EFT for WEIGHT LOSS

The Revolutionary Technique for Conquering
Emotional Overeating, Cravings, Bingeing,
Eating Disorders, and Self-Sabotage

Featuring Reports from EFT Practitioners,
Instructors, Students, and Users

by Dawson Church
www.EFTUniverse.com

Energy Psychology Press
3340 Fulton Rd., #442, Fulton, CA 95439
www.EFTUniverse.com

Cataloging-in-Publication Data

Church, Dawson, 1956–

EFT for weight loss : the revolutionary technique for conquering emotional overeating, cravings, bingeing, eating disorders, and self-sabotage / by Dawson Church — 3rd ed.

p. cm.

"Featuring reports from EFT practitioners, instructors, students, and users."
Includes index.

ISBN 978-1-60415-215-9

1. Weight loss. 2. Emotional Freedom Techniques. 3. Eating disorders—Alternative treatment. I. Title.

RM222.2.C716 2010

613.2'5—dc22

2010028365
© 2013 Dawson Church

Cover design by Victoria Valentine
Editing by CJ Puotinen and Stephanie Marohn
Typesetting by Karin Kinsey
Typeset in Cochin and Adobe Garamond
Printed in USA by Bang Printing
Third Edition

10 9 8 7 6 5 4 3 2 1

Contents

How to Use This Book

Welcome to *EFT for Weight Loss!* The book you now hold in your hands has the potential to end your years of searching for weight loss solutions. It offers you a path to easy and permanent weight loss, based on sound science and proven experience. You'll learn what it takes to apply EFT successfully in your life, eliminating cravings and behaviors that have sabotaged your previous efforts. My intention is that this is the last weight loss book you will ever need, because these methods are so effective! Here's how to use this book.

Start with the Introduction, Chapter 1, and the first section of Chapter 2: Your First Experience of Tapping for Cravings. Taken together, these sections will give you an understanding of how EFT works for weight loss (Introduction), teach you the basics of EFT (Chapter 1), and give you a powerful personal experience applying EFT to your own cravings (first section of Chapter 2).

Once you've had an experience of how effective EFT can be, start applying it regularly, and use the remaining chapters for inspiration and guidance. They contain the stories of many people just like you in the sense that they were unsuccessful with weight loss till they discovered EFT. EFT is phenomenally effective at reducing stress. Read the chapters on the topics that are most relevant to you.

Once you've been using EFT for a while, experiment with the Full Basic Recipe found in Appendix A. The version of EFT you'll learn in Chapter 2 is a shortcut, and leaves out elements of the routine found in the Full Basic Recipe. That routine is able to shift urges and negative emotions that were installed in your body and subconscious mind at a very early age. The shortcut version clears the emotional trauma at the surface, while the Full Basic Recipe can go very deep.

This book is designed as a companion to *The EFT Manual* (Church, 2013) and the materials on the EFTUniverse.com website. This website is an astonishing resource, containing the collected wisdom of the whole EFT community in the form of thousands of stories, case histories, and personal reports. On EFT Universe, you'll find cases written up by doctors, nurses, psychiatrists and psychologists, as well as thousands of stories written by ordinary people, some of whom got fantastic results the first time they tried EFT. A selection of these stories is featured in this book, but at EFT Universe you'll find thousands more, many of them about successful weight loss.

You'll make the fastest progress if you use this book in conjunction with other EFT resources. EFT Universe offers dozens of free videos designed to allow you to tap along with others. I strongly recommend taking a live EFT workshop. These workshops are taught by expert EFT trainers, and give you hands-on experience with EFT. You can also sign up for one of our online weight loss classes. We have designed a state-of-the-art, six-week program called Skinny Genes (SkinnyGenesFit.com) which cements the practices of successful weight loss in your mind and body, and has helped thousands of people to lose weight and keep it off.

With all these resources to help you on your journey, you are well supported! If you stick with the approach offered in this book, you'll have a strong likelihood of success. Though you might be tempted to give up after you binge or lapse, just get back on the program. Remember those immortal words that it's not how often you fall down that matters, but how many times you pick yourself up again. You'll feel how much I care about your success as you read these pages, use the online Skinny Genes program, and read the stories on EFT Universe. Yes, it is possible for you to lose weight and keep it off permanently, and the book you hold in your hand is your key to success.

References

Church, D. (2013). *The EFT manual* (3rd ed.). Santa Rosa, CA: Energy Psychology Press.

Introduction

I am so excited to share the information in this book with you. It's not just another diet guide, eating plan, or medical textbook. This book offers you a proven formula that has been used by thousands of people to lose weight. Those people had tried other methods, but without success. Most of them had tried many other methods, and came to EFT with a track record of failure. They were hopeful, but experience had taught them that yet another approach had a small chance of success. Against this backdrop of failure and disappointment, they began their journey of weight loss with EFT.

Hard Truths from a Nutritionist

Here's the story of Karen Donaldson, a certified nutritionist and weight loss coach who herself had trouble with weight:

"As a registered dietitian, personal trainer, and owner of a weight loss clinic, there is *lots* of pressure on me not only to help others lose weight, but for *me* to be able to lose weight and keep it off. To be honest, I'd been stuck for about ten years and my weight simply would not budge. I was lucky that I carried it well, but I was still on the heavier side. I would be good during the day, but at night I would find myself sitting in front of the television eating a huge bowl of popcorn, followed by chocolate. I would also eat very large portions of pasta and I could never have potato chips in the house! I knew other people ate for emotional reasons, but I didn't think I was one of them!

"About four years ago, I started looking for answers to help my clients and I came across EFT. As I started to share it with them, I noticed that as *they* were getting results, so was I! I was finally starting to lose weight. My cravings were decreasing and I wasn't eating as much pasta and potato chips. Over the next few years, I continued to work with EFT on myself and with my clients with amazing results. I was hooked! Using EFT and energy work, including the skills I learned in the Skinny Genes class, I've lost about twenty-five pounds—and *kept it off!* The best thing of all is that it's not hard. It's not a matter of willpower anymore. I've been working on healing my *real* issues and, as a result, my relationship with food has changed. I rarely have cravings or eat for emotional issues. I'm truly experiencing peace with food—and with life.

"As a side benefit, my relationship with my spouse has improved, as well as my relationship with myself. I love EFT and all that it has to offer. It's by far the best tool I've ever used for weight loss. And I love my job! Every day I get to help people calm their cravings and heal their emotions. Everyone should be doing EFT."

Karen's experience is common to many people. Some have lost five pounds; others have lost 105 pounds or more. Whatever your weight loss goal, EFT can help.

My Personal Story

My personal weight loss goal when I began the process was forty pounds. At that time, I was in my early fifties and I weighed around 285 pounds. Even though I'm 6 feet 5 inches tall, being over 280 meant I was obviously and perpetually fat. I'd gained the weight little by little most years, though there were several periods of my life when I was very stressed and gained a substantial amount of weight fast. One of these times was when I became the CEO of a struggling book publishing and distribution company. I was able to turn the company around and sales doubled in the first year. But in that year I gained about twenty pounds. Now, that's less than two pounds a month, which doesn't seem like a lot. Yet even that small incremental amount adds up to twenty-four pounds in the course of a single year. Multiply that by a decade, and you can see how people like you and me can find ourselves weighing a great deal more than we wish.

I was very aware that I had a problem, even when I was 250 pounds. I began to read weight loss books and magazine articles. I joined a gym and a food program. I counted calories. Each weight loss program produced temporary results, but failed in the long run. I would lose a few pounds, but they returned, and I wound up being heavier than I was before. Does that sound familiar? Virtually everyone who reads this book has a variation of this story.

Other parts of my life, other than weight, were going great. At that time I was presenting at many medical and psychology conferences each year. Speakers receive evaluations from conference attendees, and my presentations were usually ranked among the top 10 percent of all speakers. My book *The Genie in Your Genes* was a best-seller, and I founded a successful publishing company, Energy Psychology Press. My book is about epigenetics, the science of how the genes in our cells are affected by influences from outside the cell itself. Genes can be turned on or off by many external forces, and emotions are a particularly potent source controlling the process. I received many invitations to present my work to professional audiences.

Yet when I would stand up to speak, it was obvious to the whole audience that I had a problem with weight. They couldn't see the money in my bank account or the amazing ideas in my head, but they certainly could see the big spare tire I carried around my waist!

The Many Myths That Keep You Stuck

All that changed when I got serious about weight loss with EFT. I took a look at the science behind successful weight loss, and was surprised to discover that most of what I'd been told about weight loss by so-called "experts" was just plain wrong. Do you know the answers to these questions?

- Does it matter if you eat the same on weekends and weekdays?

- Which diet is best?

- After you lose weight, does keeping it off get easier or harder over time?

- Which produces fastest weight loss: diet or exercise?

- Is the importance of eating breakfast fact or myth?

- Should you weigh yourself frequently?

- If you make a slip, should you return immediately to your weight loss program?

When I began to investigate the research, I found that the field of weight loss is filled with myths, and that unfortunate people like you and me put huge amounts of energy into approaches that are ineffective. We torture our bodies and minds using unscientific strategies that are doomed to fail. Meanwhile, there are scientific answers drawn from sound research studies to the previous questions, and the approach in this book is based on these. Weight loss is actually quite simple when you toss out all the bad advice and use just a few principles that are based on clear research evidence.

EFT allowed me to make effective use of all the weight loss tools at my disposal, and I lost those forty pounds in about six months. I then kept them off for six months, after which I taught my first live weight loss class. The outline of that class eventually became part of this book and the Skinny Genes online course, which I created with EFT practitioner Brittany Watkins. As I write this introduction to this book, it's exactly three years to the month that I've been able to maintain that weight loss. Studies show that if you can maintain your weight loss for a year or more, you're highly unlikely to gain it back (Wing & Phelan, 2005). As you can see, I'm passionately committed to you being as successful as I was.

How Is EFT Different?

What makes EFT successful for people like you and me who have failed at other weight loss programs? The answer is based on several key distinctions.

First, EFT has a phenomenal ability to *reduce your cravings*. Whether you crave ice cream, chocolate, alcohol, tobacco, sweets, or anything else, EFT is able to make those cravings go away in minutes. This is not an unsupported claim; it is a scientific fact. Together with Audrey Brooks, PhD, a research psychologist at the University of Arizona, I conducted a trial of EFT that examined mental health and cravings (Church & Brooks, 2010).

We gathered data from 216 health-care professionals. These were psychotherapists, doctors, nurses, psychiatrists, alternative medicine practitioners, and chiropractors. They participated in a daylong EFT group workshop at one of five professional conferences. As part of that workshop, we examined addictive cravings for items like chocolate, food, alcohol, and tobacco in health-care workers. The declines in cravings were substantial, averaging 83 percent (p < .0001). In a separate study, we measured psychological symptoms in a group of people with self-identified craving and addiction problems attending a two-day group workshop focused on these issues. We found improvements across a spectrum of mental health conditions, including depression and anxiety (Church & Brooks, 2013).

Reducing cravings is a key manner in which EFT helps with weight loss. If your craving for that candy bar or bucket of ice cream goes away, and you don't eat it, then all those calories don't enter your body. Craving reduction is key to weight loss.

Second, EFT is able to *reduce mental health problems such as anxiety and depression.* Studies have found an association between depression and obesity. A study of 487 obese individuals found that weight loss was associated with a sustained reduction in depressive symptom levels, noting that obesity "causes or exacerbates depression" (Wing & Phelan, 2005, p. 2058). Obese people tend to have higher levels of depression, and depressed people tend to have higher levels of obesity. This is not surprising, because being fat is depressing!

Depression levels are a predictor of how likely it is that you will regain weight after dieting (McGuire, Wing, Klem, Lang, & Hill, 1999). Depression decreases the likelihood that you will keep that weight off even if you succeed in losing it. That's even more depressing!

Being fat is also a very obvious problem that you carry around with you every day. Other problems might not be obvious to outsiders. You can meet a person who looks good, but is going through a miserable time in some part of their life. Yet you don't know it from the outside. Problems like financial failure, divorce, and spiritual poverty don't show up in the same way as obesity does. If you're overweight, everyone knows immediately, while if a person is failing in some other area of their life, their body doesn't advertise it in the form of flab. Speaking from experience, it's depressing to be dragging your problem pounds around for everyone to see. Your failure to maintain your weight is obvious to anyone the second they meet you.

In another cruel twist of reality, your failure is obvious, but your success is invisible. I have a friend who recently lost thirty pounds. But she still has another fifty to go, and all people see now is the fifty she has to go, not the thirty she's already lost. All her hard work, consistency, discipline, and focus that resulted in weight loss is completely unappreciated by anyone other than her friends. Strangers only see her failure, and cannot appreciate her success. That's also depressing.

Many studies have found big drops in depressive symptom levels after EFT (Church, 2013a). Whether depression is studied in veterans with PTSD, college students, or dieters, they all improve. By improving your mental health, EFT makes it much more likely that your improvements will stick.

Third, EFT helps with *emotional eating*. Clinical psychologist Roger Callahan, PhD, who developed one of the earliest methods on which EFT is based, observed that cravings usually mask anxiety (Callahan, 2000). Below the craving is anxiety, and we eat to suppress that anxiety.

There's a Japanese story about two groups of disciples of two different spiritual masters. They were having a fierce argument about whose master was the most advanced. The disciples of one group presented their evidence that theirs was truly an adept: He could fly through the air, turn base metal into gold, and read minds. The disciples of the other group laughed, and said their master demonstrated even greater accomplishments. The first group was flabbergasted. What on earth could the second master do that would eclipse those accomplishments, they demanded. Here's what the second master's students said: He sleeps when he's tired. He drinks when he's thirsty. He eats when he's hungry.

Their point was that he'd mastered simply being in a body, and living in a balanced manner. Those of us who are obese or overweight cannot make that claim. Roughly a third of those living in the Northern Hemisphere are obese, and another third are overweight. That means that two-thirds of the population has not mastered the skill of eating and drinking in a way that allows us to maintain a stable balanced healthy weight.

We eat for many reasons other than hunger. We eat when we're nervous. We eat when we're lonely. We eat when we're depressed. We eat to reduce stress. We eat to reward ourselves. We eat to mask our feelings. None of these emotional reasons for eating has anything to do with the body's need for nourishment. This disconnect between the act of eating and the body's requirements for sustenance is characteristic of many people. We might have even lost touch with our body's signals that it's had enough food, or that it doesn't like some of the junk we're shoving down our throats. Our emotions are overriding our body's signals. That's the problem with emotional eating, and EFT has a proven ability to help reduce the trauma that is the source of so much negative emotion.

What Is EFT?

EFT is also called "tapping" because a central practice of EFT is to use your fingertips to tap lightly on points on your body. These points are described in the ancient Oriental technique of acupuncture. Acupuncture points are spots on energy meridians that flow through your body. They conduct energy well, having only about 1/2000th the electromagnetic resistance found in the surrounding skin (Hyvarien & Karlson, 1977).

While you tap, you think about events or beliefs that bothered you. Perhaps one day when you were six years old, your ten-year-old brother called you "Fattie" in front of his best friend Bruce. You had a crush on Bruce, and you felt humiliated. Another time, when you were twelve, your mother took you to a store to buy a new outfit, and the clerk sneered and said, "I don't think we have anything in her size." You tried out for a part in the school play when you were fourteen, and the drama teacher condescendingly declared, "You aren't the right shape for this role." By the time you're an adult, you have a large collection of these events contributing to your anxiety and depression, along with many failed attempts at dieting. You've developed a poor self-image and have a toxic collection of memories in your mind. The voices of fear and self-doubt whisper in your ear every time you try and solve your problems.

EFT trains you to tap on each of these formative experiences. Tapping sends soothing signals throughout your body. When you tap while remembering bad events, the emotional intensity of the bad events evaporates. You still remember them, but they are no longer filled with an emotional charge (Church, 2013b).

As you remember them and tap, EFT also has you say words of comfort and self-affirmation, like "I deeply and completely accept myself." Remembering a painful memory + tapping + self-affirmation is the secret sauce. Tapping and self-affirmation remove the sting from the memory. After EFT, you might occasionally recall the memory, but it's no longer loaded with emotional baggage. Your past hasn't changed, but the lens through which you see it is neural, instead of being overlaid with anger, shame, sorrow, blame, and guilt.

There's a huge amount of science behind EFT, but, in a nutshell, that's the effect it has. Let's take a look at just a piece of that scientific research, and see what happens when people like you and me use EFT for weight loss.

Hormones and Science

There's a great deal of research into EFT, so much so that it's considered an "evidence-based" practice (Church, 2013a). You can read about it at the research bibliography at EFT Universe, but I'd like to highlight a few studies that show how powerfully it can help you with weight loss as well as your mental health.

A colleague of mine, Peta Stapleton, a professor at Bond University, conducted a randomized controlled trial of EFT in a group of ninety-six weight loss subjects (Stapleton, Sheldon, Porter, & Whitty, 2011). She found that their levels of restraint increased after EFT in comparison to a control group. Restraint is important because it stops people from taking actions like eating too much that they later regret. The power food held over the participants decreased after EFT, indicating that they were more in control, rather than food itself dictating their actions.

If we see improvements in psychological symptoms such as anxiety and depression after EFT, as well as improvements in restraint and control, what's happening to the hormones of those people? Over the last decade, I've been fascinated by the stress hormone cortisol and began studying the link between EFT and cortisol.

Research has shown a link between levels of cortisol and both depression and obesity. High cortisol levels are linked to the accumulation of fatty adipose tissue around the midsection of the body (Björntorp, 2001). Depression is also associated with elevated cortisol (Holsboer, 2000). These studies also show that high cortisol and depression are associated with many different forms of ill health, including high blood pressure, poor metabolism, high cholesterol, and poor regulation of insulin.

Along with two colleagues, Audrey Brooks, PhD, and molecular biologist Garret Yount, PhD, of the California Pacific Research Institute, I performed a study that looked at cortisol before and after an EFT session (Church, Yount, & Brooks, 2012). We used a large group, eighty-three people, and randomized them into one of three treatments. A third got a session of EFT, another third received regular talk therapy, while the final group rested in one of the five clinics in which we performed the trials.

The results were striking. Anxiety and depression symptoms declined by twice as much in the EFT group as in the talk therapy group. Cortisol levels also went down much more: a 24 percent reduction in ninety minutes. That's a huge drop. What seems to be happening is that, as we feel better, with EFT reducing anxiety and depression, our fat-generating hormone cortisol declines. As we dump the stress, we dump the hormones needed to drive stress. That can help with weight loss.

Peta Stapleton and I also looked at the depression levels in her subjects, and found that they declined significantly (Stapleton, Church, Sheldon, Porter, & Carlopio, 2013). Along with EFT reducing cortisol, it's clearly reducing depression. Using EFT pays dividends in both our stress hormone levels and our mental health.

You don't have to meet with a coach or therapist in an office session to receive benefit from using EFT. It works over the phone (Hartung & Stein, 2011) and over the Internet (Brattberg, 2008). The 2008 study by physician Gunilla Brattberg, MD, was particularly interesting because she offered EFT as an online therapy only; participants never talked to a doctor or psychotherapist. Yet their depressive symptoms declined significantly. This has led to the development of other Internet-based methods of offering EFT for a variety of problems including post-traumatic stress disorder (PTSD) and weight loss.

We used the introduction of the Skinny Genes online weight loss course as an opportunity to conduct a clinical trial of online EFT. The results were very encouraging. Over the course of the six-week program, participants lost an average of twelve pounds (Church & Wilde, 2013). That averages out as two pounds a week, which most medical authorities regard as a safe and steady level, rather than the precipitous weight loss advocated by more extreme programs.

The bottom line of all this research into EFT is that it improves both mental and physical health. There's no clear dividing line between the mind and the body, so as your mental health improves, your physical health tags right along, and vice versa. The side benefit of better mental health is better physical health.

Characteristics of Long-Term Weight Loss

One of the persistent problems with diets is that they're usually futile in the long run. Sure, dieters lose weight, but after the diet most of them gain it all back. Not so with EFT! Studies of people who take an EFT course for weight loss show that they continue to lose weight after the course ends. Stapleton, Sheldon, and Porter (2012) found that in the year following their weight loss program, participants lost an additional eleven pounds on average.

I also took a look at the amount of weight loss that occurred after people completed the Skinny Genes program, knowing that temporary weight loss was not worth the effort. Our clinical trial showed that Skinny Genes participants lost an average of three pounds in the six months following the Skinny Genes online program (Church & Wilde, 2013). Skinny Genes does not focus on weight loss per se, nor prescribe any particular diet, but instead focuses on the emotional aspects of eating. We believe that once emotional eating goes away, weight loss follows naturally. A friend of mine recently began tapping on all his memories on the theme of "shame." He'd had many events in his life that contributed to the theme, and he tapped on them one by one. A few weeks after starting the process, he told me, with wonder in his voice, that thirty pounds had simply melted away. It wasn't physical; the weight was emotional. When he dealt with the emotional events, the weight dropped away.

While it's true that most dieters eventually gain back all the weight they lost, and more, it's not true of everyone. A small percentage of dieters are successful at losing weight and keeping it off for good. A database maintained by the National Weight Control Registry shows that 20 percent of individuals who lose 10 percent or more of their body weight keep it off for a year or more (Wing &

Phelan, 2005). It's well worth taking a close look at how they were successful, and emulating them, helped by EFT. What is it these people do that makes them successful? They demonstrate six primary characteristics:

1. They weigh themselves frequently. They monitor themselves regularly, so that they can correct their course as soon as they stray. The reason this is important is that it establishes a feedback loop between what you eat and what you weigh. When you eat that bowl of ice cream, weigh yourself the following morning, and see that you've gained a pound, you understand the link between the two events. When you stick with your diet all weekend and notice on Monday morning that you've lost two pounds, you associate the two. Over time, you take a look at what you're eating and evaluate it in terms of how much weight you'll gain or lose if you put it in your mouth. You still have a choice, but now you understand the consequences of those choices. Write down your weight in a journal every day after you weigh yourself. This way, you'll also start to notice patterns. The registry found that 75 percent of participants weigh themselves at least once a week, and most of these weigh themselves once a day.

2. They maintain their eating habits each day. They don't indulge on weekends and fast on weekdays, or eat excessively during the holiday season and starve themselves afterward. Their bodies are treated to a nice even baseline of ingredients. They've discovered what works for weight maintenance, and they stick to it.

3. They exercise regularly. Exercise isn't key to weight loss in the way diet is, but exercise is vital to health. Those in the study exercised an average of an hour a day. That exercise doesn't have to be pumping iron in the gym or running on the treadmill; even moderate exercise like thirty minutes of walking each day has been shown to help nudge gene expression in a healthy direction (Ornish et al., 2008). Very few people in the registry used exercise only for weight loss (1%), and other studies have shown that diet is much more effective than exercise for weight loss. That said, exercise helps keep you healthy, and it's a habit of those who lose weight and keep it off. A predominance of the people in the registry (89%) said they used a combination of exercise and diet to keep their weight down.

4. They eat breakfast. An examination of the data from successful long-term weight loss participants shows that almost 80 percent of them eat breakfast daily; many experts consider it one of the foundations of a successful weight-loss program.

5. They eat a diet that is low in calories and fat. They watch their food intake carefully, with 88 percent of them restricting foods they know make them fat. Many (43%) count calories, even two or three years after they've lost weight. Vigilance keeps them skinny.

6. Whenever they slip, they catch themselves quickly. Data from the registry show that people who slip and don't correct quickly are a lot more likely to gain weight than those that do. Successful long-term

weight losers notice when they've gained weight, identify what happened to produce that result, and return as fast as possible to their baseline habits. Over half of the people in the registry (55%) are still focused on losing weight and are not casual about their success.

Right at the start of your weight loss program, keep these six behaviors in mind. At the back of this book, you'll find two pages you can copy and post where you see them daily. One is "EFT on a Page." The other is "Tapping Plan for Weight Loss." Copy these pages and pin them up in your house. Post them on your refrigerator. Make copies and paste them *inside* your refrigerator! Put another copy inside your freezer, one in your wallet, one on your bathroom mirror. Consider these six tips the advice you've received from people who've succeeded and are eager to help you succeed too. They've achieved the goal; we've studied how they accomplished it, and we're making their secret formula available to you through this book and through the Skinny Genes program.

How To Use EFT with These Principles

You'll learn a lot about how to use EFT in this book, and it fits neatly into the principles just outlined. You can use EFT to help with each of these practices, as well as for much more, such as reducing cravings and eliminating emotional eating. Here's how EFT fits into your weight loss routine.

1. Tap on any resistance that arises in your mind or emotions around the habits and goals you've set

yourself. For instance, you might have set yourself a goal of joining a gym, but three years have gone by and somehow you haven't quite gotten around to it. Or you've committed to cutting "empty calories" from your diet, but they somehow find their way into your grocery cart every time you shop. Or you know you ought to buy a scale, but somehow you "forget" every time you visit the store. Perhaps you know you ought to eat breakfast every day, but you realize around noon each day that it's slipped your mind. The reason that your behavior doesn't reflect your goals is that part of you is resisting the changes you'd like to make. EFT is great at eliminating such resistance. In the coming chapters, we show you exactly how to do this.

2. Tap on body sensations. When you sit down with a plate of food, what signals is your body giving you? How do you know which foods your body really doesn't want (even though other parts of you do)? Are you aware of exactly how your body signals you when it is full? Tapping while tuning in to body sensations puts you in tune with your body, and makes you sensitive to what it's trying to tell you. You develop a natural sensitivity to its signals. These become a guide to healthy behavior and weight.

3. Tap on emotions that arise while eating and around food. What do you feel when you view a plate of your favorite food? Your least favorite food? A big portion? A small portion? A list of healthy foods? A list of forbidden foods? When you're hungry? When you're full? In the snack aisle of the supermarket?

In the vegetable aisle? When you eat fast? When you eat slowly? As you start to use EFT, you'll find that an enormous part of your reaction to food is not physical at all but, rather, emotional. When we "tap away" these emotional responses, we begin to hear the real language of our body that has been drowned out by emotional triggers.

You'll also tap on emotions that arise around the topic of eating consistently. If you feel deprived on Friday afternoon because you're used to bingeing on the weekends, you'll tap on that. You can also tap as you contemplate high-fat, high-calorie foods you know will pack on the pounds. Just tap while looking at them. You'll find that the emotional attraction to those foods can rapidly disappear as you tap.

When you slip up in your diet and exercise regimen, EFT is great at offering you self-acceptance. Rather than reinforcing self-recrimination about your lapse, EFT reminds you to accept yourself. It refocuses you on the big picture of self-acceptance rather than staying in a place of beating yourself up about your lapse.

4. Reinforce your intentions by tapping. Perhaps you're going to a party, and you know you'll be tempted by the foods that are your downfall, that have packed on the weight in the past. Before you leave for the party, you can imagine being there, tapping along while you vividly picture your temptations. Maybe the holidays are coming up, and you know you always gain weight. Imagine yourself going right through

the holidays, frame by frame, and sticking to sensible portions. Visualize yourself passing up the opportunities to binge; tapping will reinforce your intentions, setting you up for success.

5. Throughout this book, I'm going to have you do a great deal of tapping on adverse events that occurred during your childhood that might contribute to overeating. You might not be too keen on revisiting those bad experience, but please trust me on this: Horrible though they might be when you remember them today, your emotional triggering will rapidly diminish when you use EFT. You'll be surprised at how fast events that bother you to the max today lose their sting in minutes with EFT. This seems like magic, but there's a lot of science to explain how EFT works so quickly.

6. Tap on your objections to success. I'm going to help you find core beliefs and inner messages that are obstructing your forward movement. These hidden objections to success might be buried deep in your subconscious mind. EFT includes several powerful techniques that bring these hidden beliefs to light. Once you're aware of them, you can un-install them by tapping.

How I Applied the Principles

When I began weighing myself every day, and recording my weight in my journal, as recommended by the National Weight Control Registry, I noticed a pattern. Every time I went on a speaking trip, I gained about five pounds. The reason was not hard to find. Out of my home environment, I was eating at restaurants, with limited choices. A chicken romaine salad that was low calorie at home was high calorie on the road. A restaurant might serve it smothered in rich Caesar dressing, tripling the number of calories in the dish. Meals on the road, such as a continental breakfast, were often high in simple carbohydrates, which pack weight onto our bodies, and low on lean protein, which are packed with energy while being low in calories.

I also noticed that whenever I ate foods packed with "empty calories," such as bread, pasta, potatoes, rice, cake, and other simple carbohydrates, the scale told me the next day that I had gained a pound or two.

Does that mean that I never eat these? No! I love pasta, and sometimes I eat it with great enjoyment. But I eat in moderation, knowing that too much today will add pounds to the scale tomorrow.

Sometimes I tap while eating a meal. I notice what emotions arise in my body as I look at, taste, touch, and smell the food. I enjoy the meal just as much, but I've noticed I'm less likely to clean my plate if I'm tapping. I also imagine dangerous situations in which I know I'll be tempted to overeat, and I tap in advance.

I've also uncovered many unhealthy and painful early experiences around eating and food, and tapped away the emotional intensity behind them.

As I've done this, my whole relationship to food has changed. I enjoy tasting it much more; it's now my friend rather than my enemy. I've come into greater harmony with my body. I believe I've slowed the aging process; certainly, dragging forty fewer pounds around each day makes my life much easier. My legs thank me, and my back thanks me. I have a congenital spinal deformity that predisposes me to back pain, and I've had much less pain now that I'm no longer carrying all those superfluous pounds. I look better and feel better.

You'll find dozens of other tips from EFT experts in the pages of this book. The final chapter ties it all together by giving you a detailed and specific Tapping Plan for Weight Loss. This plan includes all the behaviors you can practice to lose weight and keep it off. Though they take just a few minutes each day, research shows that if you use them, you're likely to find the success that has eluded you up till now.

As you can tell, I'm passionate about sharing these discoveries with you. Please stick to this program, and you might well surprise yourself by how fast you make progress.

References

Brattberg, G. (2008). Self-administered EFT (Emotional Freedom Techniques) in individuals with fibromyalgia: A randomized trial. *Integrative Medicine: A Clinician's Journal, 7*(4), 30–35.

Björntorp, P. (2001). Do stress reactions cause abdominal obesity and comorbidities?. *Obesity Reviews, 2*(2), 73–86.

Callahan, R. (2000). *Tapping the healer within: Using Thought Field Therapy to instantly conquer your fears, anxieties, and emotional distress.* New York: McGraw-Hill.

Church, D. (2013a). Clinical EFT as an evidence-based practice for the treatment of psychological and physiological conditions. *Psychology* (in press).

Church, D. (2013b). *The EFT manual* (3rd ed.). Santa Rosa, CA: Energy Psychology Press.

Church, D., & Brooks, A. J. (2010). The effect of a brief EFT (Emotional Freedom Techniques) self-intervention on anxiety, depression, pain and cravings in healthcare workers. *Integrative Medicine: A Clinician's Journal, 9*(4), 40–44.

Church, D., & Brooks, A. J. (2013). The Effect of EFT (Emotional Freedom Techniques) on psychological symptoms in addiction treatment: A pilot study. *International Journal of Scientific Research and Reports* (in press).

Church, D. & Wilde, N. (2013, May). Emotional eating and weight loss following Skinny Genes, a six week online program. Reported at the annual conference of Association for Comprehensive Energy Psychology (ACEP), Reston, VA.

Church, D., Yount, G., & Brooks, A. J. (2012). The effect of Emotional Freedom Techniques (EFT) on stress biochemistry: A randomized controlled trial. *Journal of Nervous and Mental Disease, 200,* 891–896. doi:10.1097/NMD.0b013e31826b9fc1

Hartung, J., & Stein, P. (2011). Telephone delivery of EFT remediates PTSD symptoms in veterans: A randomized controlled trial. *Energy Psychology: Theory, Research, and Treatment, 4*(1), 33–40.

Holsboer, F. (2000). The corticosteroid receptor hypothesis of depression. *Neuropsychopharmacology, 23*(5), 477–501.

Hyvarien, J. & Karlson, M. (1977). Low resistance skin points that may coincide with acupuncture locations. *Medical Biology*, *55*, 88–94.

McGuire, M. T., Wing, R. R., Klem, M. L., & Hill, J. O. (1999) What predicts weight regain in a group of successful weight losers? *Journal of Consulting and Clinical Psychology*, *67*(2),177–185.

Ornish, D., Magbanua, M. J. M., Weidner, G., Weinberg, V., Kemp, C., Green, C., et al. (2008). Changes in prostate gene expression in men undergoing an intensive nutrition and lifestyle intervention. *Proceedings of the National Academy of Sciences USA*, *105*(24), 8369–8374.

Stapleton, P., Church, D., Sheldon, T., Porter, B., & Carlopio, C. (2013). Depression symptoms improve after successful weight loss with EFT (Emotional Freedom Techniques): A randomized controlled trial. *Psychiatry* (in press).

Stapleton, P., Sheldon, T., Porter, B., & Whitty, J. (2011). A randomised clinical trial of a meridian-based intervention for food cravings with six-month follow-up. *Behaviour Change*, *28*(1), 1.

Stapleton, P. B., Sheldon, T., & Porter, B. (2012). Clinical benefits of Emotional Freedom Techniques on food cravings at 12-months follow-up: A randomized controlled trial. *Energy Psychology: Theory, Research, and Treatment*, *4*(1), 1–12.

Wing, R. R., & Phelan, S. (2005). Long-term weight loss maintenance. *American Journal of Clinical Nutrition*, *82*, 222–225.

1

EFT's Basic Recipe

Over the past decade, EFT has been the focus of a great deal of research. This has resulted in more than twenty clinical trials, in which EFT has been demonstrated to reduce a wide variety of symptoms. These include pain, skin rashes, fibromyalgia, depression, anxiety, and posttraumatic stress disorder (PTSD). Most of these studies have used the standardized form of EFT found in *The EFT Manual.* In this chapter, my goal is to show you how to unlock EFTs healing benefits from whatever physical or psychological problems you're facing. I have a passionate interest in relieving human suffering. When you study EFT, you quickly realize how much suffering can be alleviated with the help of this extraordinary healing tool. I'd like to place the full power of that tool in your hands, so that you can live the happiest, healthiest, and most abundant life possible.

If you go on YouTube or do a Google search, you will find thousands of websites and videos about EFT. The quality of the EFT information you'll find through these sources varies widely, however. Certified practitioners trained in EFT provide a small portion of the information. Most of it consists of personal testimonials by untrained enthusiasts. It's great that EFT works to some degree for virtually anyone. To get the most out of EFT and unlock its full potential, however, it's essential that you learn the form of EFT that's been proven in so many clinical trials. We call this Clinical EFT.

Every year in EFT Universe workshops, we get many people who tell us variations of the same story: "I saw a video on YouTube, tapped along, and got amazing results the first few times. Then it seemed to stop working." The reason for this is that a superficial application of EFT can indeed work wonders. To unleash the full power of EFT, however, requires learning the standardized form we call Clinical EFT, which has been validated, over and over again, by high-quality research, and is taught systematically, step by step, by top experts, in EFT workshops.

Why is EFT able to affect so many problems, both psychological and physical? The reason for its effectiveness is that it reduces stress, and stress is a component of many problems. In EFT research on pain, for instance, we find that pain decreases by an average of 68 percent with EFT. That's a two-thirds drop, and seems very impressive. Now ask yourself, if EFT can produce a two-thirds drop in pain, why can't it produce a 100 percent drop? I pondered this question myself, and I asked many therapists and doctors for their theories as to why this might be so.

The consensus is that the two-thirds of pain reduced by EFT is due largely to emotional causes, while the remaining one-third of the pain has a physical derivation. A man I'll call "John" volunteered for a demonstration at an EFT introductory evening at which I presented. He was on crutches, and told us he had a broken leg as a result of a car accident. On a scale of 0 to 10, with 0 being no pain, and 10 being maximum pain, he rated his pain as an 8. The accident had occurred two weeks earlier. My logical scientific brain didn't think EFT would work for John, because his pain was purely physical. I tapped with him anyway. At the end of our session, which lasted less than 15 minutes, his pain was down to a 2. I hadn't tapped on the actual pain with John at all, but rather on all the emotional components of the auto accident.

There were many such components. His wife had urged him to drive to an event, but he didn't want to go. He had resentment toward his wife. That's emotional. He was angry at the driver of the other car. That's emotional. He was mad at himself for abandoning his own needs by driving to an event he didn't want to attend. That's emotional. He was upset that now, as an adult, he was reenacting the abandonment he experienced by his mother when he was a child. That's emotional. He was still hurt by an incident that occurred when he was five years old, when his mother was supposed to pick him up from a friend's birthday party and forgot because she was socializing with her friends and drinking. That's emotional.

Do you see the pattern here? We're working on a host of problems that are emotional, yet interwoven with the pain. The physical pain is overlaid with a matrix of emotional issues, like self-neglect, abandonment, anger, and frustration, which are part of the entire fabric of John's life.

The story has a happy ending. After we'd tapped on each of these emotional components of John's pain, the physical pain in his broken leg went down to a 2. That pain rating revealed the extent of the physical component of John's problem. It was a 2. The other six points were emotional.

The same is true for the person who's afraid of public speaking, who has a spider phobia, who's suffering from a physical ailment, who's feeling trapped in his job, who's unhappy with her husband, who's in conflict with those around him. All of these problems have a large component of unfinished emotional business from the past. When you neutralize the underlying emotional issues with EFT, what remains is the real problem, which is often far smaller than you imagine.

Though I present at few conferences nowadays because of other demands on my time, I used to present at about thirty medical and psychological conferences each year, speaking about research and teaching EFT. I presented to thousands of medical professionals during that period. One of my favorite sayings was "Don't medicalize emotional problems. And don't emotionalize medical problems." When I would say this to a roomful of physicians, they would nod their heads in unison. The medical profession as a whole is very aware of the emotional component of disease.

If you have a real medical problem, you need good medical care. No ifs, ands, or buts. If you have an emotional problem, you need EFT. Most problems are a mixture of both. That's why I urge you to work on the emotional component with EFT and other safe and non-invasive behavioral methods, and to get the best possible medical care for the physical component of your problem. Talk to your doctor about this; virtually every physician will be supportive of you bolstering your medical treatment with emotional catharsis.

When you feel better emotionally, a host of positive changes also occur in your energy system. When you feel worse, your energy system follows. Several researchers have hooked people up to electroencephalographs (EEGs), and taken EEG readings of the electrical energy in their brains before and after EFT. These studies show that when subjects are asked to recall a traumatic event, their patterns of brain-wave activity change. The brain-wave frequencies associated with stress, and activation of the fight-or-flight response, dominate their EEG readings. After successful treatment, the brain waves shown on their EEG readings are those that characterize relaxation.

Other research has shown similar results from acupuncture. The theory behind acupuncture is that our body's energy flows in twelve channels called meridians. When that energy is blocked, physical or psychological distress occurs. The use of acupuncture needles, or acupressure with the fingertips, is believed to release those energy blocks. EFT has you tap with your fingertips on the end points of those meridians; that's why it's sometimes called "emotional acupuncture." When your energy is balanced and flowing, whether it's the brain-wave energy picked up by the EEG or the meridian energy described in acupuncture, you feel better. That's another reason why EFT works well for many different kinds of problem.

EFT is rooted in sound science, and this chapter is devoted to showing you how to do Clinical EFT yourself. It will introduce you to the basic concepts that amplify the power of EFT, and steer you clear of the most common pitfalls that prevent people from making progress with EFT. The basics of EFT are easy to use and quick to learn. We call this EFT's "Basic Recipe." The second half of this chapter shows you how to apply the Basic Recipe for maximum effect. It introduces you to all of the concepts key to Clinical EFT.

Testing

EFT doesn't just hope to be effective. We test our results constantly, to determine if the course we're taking is truly making us feel better. The basic scale we use for testing was developed by a famous psychiatrist called Joseph Wolpe in the 1950s, and measures our degree of discomfort on a scale of 0 through 10. Zero indicates no discomfort, and 10 is the maximum possible distress. This scale works equally well for psychological problems such as anxiety and physical problems such as pain.

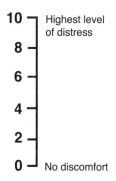

SUD scale (intensity meter)

Dr. Wolpe called this rating SUD or Subjective Units of Discomfort. It's also sometimes called Subjective Units of Distress. You feel your problem, and give it a number on the SUD scale. It's vital to rate your SUD level as it is *right now,* not imagine what it might have been at the time in the past when the traumatic event occurred. If you can't quickly identify a number, just take your best guess, and go from there.

I recommend you write down your initial SUD number. It's also worth noting *where in your body* the information on your SUD level is coming from. If you're working on a physical pain such as a headache, where in your head is the ache centered? If you're working on a traumatic emotional event, perhaps a car accident, where in your body is your reference point for your emotional distress? Do you feel it in your belly, your heart, your forehead? Write down the location on which your SUD is based.

A variation of the numeric scale is a visual scale. For example, if you're working with a child who does not yet know how to count, you can ask the child to spread his or her hands apart to indicate how big the problem is. Wide-open arms means big, and hands close together means small.

Whatever means you use to test, each round of EFT tapping usually begins with this type of assessment of the size of the problem. This allows us to determine whether or not our approach is working. After we've tested and written down our SUD level and body location, we move on to EFTs Basic Recipe. It has this name to indicate that EFT consists of certain ingredients, and if you want to be successful, you need to include them, just the way you need to include all the ingredients in a recipe for chocolate chip cookies if you want your end product to be tasty.

Many years ago I published a book by Wally Amos. Wally is better known as "Famous Amos" for his brand of chocolate chip cookies. One day I asked Wally, "Where did you get your recipe?" I thought he was going to tell me how he'd experimented with hundreds of variations to find the best possible combination of ingredients. I imagined Wally like Thomas Edison in his laboratory, obsessively combining pinches of this and smidgeons of that, year after year, in order to perfect the flavor of his cookies, the way Edison tried thousands of combinations before discovering the incandescent light bulb.

Wally's offhand response was, "I used the recipe on the back of a pack of Toll House chocolate chips." Toll House is one of the most popular brands, selling millions of packages each year, and the simple recipe is available to everyone. I was astonished, and laughed at how different the reality was from my imaginary picture of Wally as Edison. Yet the message is simple: Don't reinvent the wheel. If it works, it works. Toll House is so popular because their recipe works. Clinical EFT produces such good results because the Basic Recipe works. While a master chef might be experienced enough to produce exquisite variations, a beginner can bake excellent cookies, and get consistently great results, just by following the basic recipe. This chapter is designed to provide you with that simple yet reliable level of knowledge.

EFTs Basic Recipe omits a procedure that was part of the earliest forms of EFT, called the 9 Gamut Procedure. Though the 9 Gamut Procedure has great value for certain conditions, it isn't always necessary, so we leave it out. The version of EFT that includes it is called the Full Basic Recipe (see Appendix A of *The EFT Manual*).

The Setup Statement

The Setup Statement systematically "sets up" the problem you want to work on. Think about arranging dominoes in a line in the game of creating a chain reaction. Before you start the game, you set them up. The object of the game is to knock them down, just the way EFT expects to knock down your SUD level, but to start with, you set up the pieces of the problem.

The Setup Statement has its roots in two schools of psychology. One is called cognitive therapy, and the other is called exposure therapy. Cognitive therapy considers the large realm of your cognitions—your thoughts, beliefs, ways of relating to others, and the mental frames through which you perceive the world and your experiences.

Exposure therapy is a successful branch of psychotherapy that vividly exposes you to your negative experiences. Rather than avoiding them, you're confronted by them, with the goal of breaking your conditioned fear response to the event.

We won't go deeper into these two forms of therapy now, but you'll later see how EFT's Setup Statement draws from cognitive and exposure approaches to form a powerful combination with acupressure or tapping.

Psychological Reversal

The term Psychological Reversal is taken from energy therapies. It refers to the concept that when your energies are blocked or reversed, you develop symptoms. If you put the batteries into a flashlight backward, with the positive end where the negative should be, the light won't shine. The human body also has a polarity (see illustration). A reversal of normal polarity will block the flow of energy through the body. In acupuncture, the goal of treatment is to remove obstructions, and to allow the free flow of energy through the twelve meridians. If reversal occurs, it impedes the healing process.

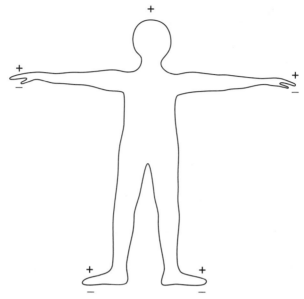

The human body's electrical polarity (adapted from
ACEP Certification Program Manual, 2006)

The way Psychological Reversal shows up in EFT and other energy therapies is as a failure to make progress in resolving the problem. It's especially prevalent in chronic diseases, addictions, and conditions that resist healing. If you run into a person who's desperate to recover, yet who has had no success even with a wide variety of different therapies, the chances are good that you're dealing with Psychological Reversal. One of the first steps of EFTs Basic Recipe is to correct for Psychological Reversal. It only takes a few seconds, so we include this step whether or not Psychological Reversal is present.

EFTs Setup includes stating an affirmation with those elements drawn from cognitive and exposure therapies, while at the same time correcting for Psychological Reversal.

Affirmation

The exposure part of the Setup Statement involves remembering the problem. You expose your mind repeatedly to the memory of the trauma. This is the opposite of what we normally do; we usually want an emotional trauma to fade away. We might engage in behaviors like dissociation or avoidance so that we don't have to deal with unpleasant memories.

As you gain confidence with EFT, you'll find yourself becoming fearless when it comes to exposure. You'll discover you don't have to remain afraid of old traumatic memories; you have a tool that allows you to reduce their emotional intensity in minutes or even seconds. The usual pattern of running away from a problem is reversed. You feel confident running toward it, knowing that you'll quickly feel better.

The EFT Setup Statement is this: *Even though I have (name of problem), I deeply and completely accept myself.*

You insert the name of the problem in the exposure half of the Setup Statement. Examples might be:

Even though I had that dreadful car crash, I deeply and completely accept myself.

Even though I have this migraine headache, I deeply and completely accept myself.

Even though I have this fear of heights, I deeply and completely accept myself.

Even though I have this pain in my knees, I deeply and completely accept myself.

Even though I had my buddy die in my arms in Iraq, I deeply and completely accept myself.

Even though I have this huge craving for whiskey, I deeply and completely accept myself.

Even though I have this fear of spiders, I deeply and completely accept myself.

Even though I have this urge to eat another cookie, I deeply and completely accept myself.

The list of variations is infinite. You can use this Setup Statement for anything that bothers you.

While exposure is represented by the first half of the Setup Statement, before the comma, cognitive work is done by the second half of the statement, the part that deals with self-acceptance. EFT doesn't try to induce you to positive thinking. You don't tell yourself that things will get better, or that you'll improve. You simply express the intention of accepting yourself just the way you are. You accept reality. Gestalt therapist Byron Katie wrote a book entitled *Loving What Is,* and that's exactly what EFT recommends you do.

The Serenity Prayer uses the same formula of acceptance, with the words, "God grant me the serenity to accept the things I cannot change; courage to change the things I can; and wisdom to know the difference." With EFT you don't try and think positively. You don't try and change your attitude or circumstances; you simply affirm that you accept them. This cognitive frame of accepting what is opens the path to change in a profound way. It's also quite difficult to do this in our culture, which bombards us with positive thinking. Positive thinking actually gets in the way of healing in many cases, while acceptance provides us with a reality-based starting point congruent with our experience. The great twentieth-century therapist Carl Rogers, who introduced client-centered therapy, said that the paradox of transformation is that change begins by accepting conditions exactly the way they are.

I recommend that you use the Setup Statement in exactly this way at first, but as you gain confidence, you can experiment with different variations. The only requirement is that you include both a self-acceptance statement and exposure to the problem. For instance, you can invert the two halves of the formula, and put cognitive self-acceptance first, followed by exposure. Here are some examples:

I accept myself fully and completely, even with this miserable headache.

I deeply love myself, even though I have nightmares from that terrible car crash.

I hold myself in high esteem, even though I feel such pain from my divorce.

When you're doing EFT with children, you don't need an elaborate Setup Statement. You can have children use very simple self-acceptance phrases, like "I'm okay" or "I'm a great kid." Such a Setup Statement might look like this:

> *Even though Johnny hit me, I'm okay.*
>
> *The teacher was mean to me, but I'm still an amazing kid.*

You'll be surprised how quickly children respond to EFT. Their SUD levels usually drop so fast that adults have a difficult time accepting the shift. Although we haven't yet done the research to discover why children are so receptive to change, my hypothesis is that their behaviors haven't yet been cemented by years of conditioning. They've not yet woven a thick neural grid in their brains through repetitive thinking and behavior, so they can let go of negative emotions fast.

What do you do if your problem is self-acceptance itself? What if you believe you're unacceptable? What if you have low self-esteem, and the words "I deeply and completely accept myself" sound like a lie?

What EFT suggests you do in such a case is say the words anyway, even if you don't believe them. They will usually have some effect, even if at first you have difficulty with them. As you correct for Psychological Reversal in the way I will show you here, you will soon find yourself shifting from unbelief to belief that you are acceptable. You can say the affirmation aloud or silently. It carries more emotional energy if it is said emphatically or loudly, and imagined vividly.

Secondary Gain

While energy therapies use the term "psychological reversal" to indicate energy blocks to healing, there's an equivalent term drawn from psychology. That term is "secondary gain." It refers to the benefits of being sick. "Why would anyone want to be sick?" you might wonder. There are actually many reasons for keeping a mental or physical problem firmly in place.

Consider the case of a veteran with PTSD. He's suffering from flashbacks of scenes from Afghanistan where he witnessed death and suffering. He has nightmares, and never sleeps through the night. He's so disturbed that he cannot hold down a job or keep a relationship intact for long. Why would such a person not want to get better, considering the damage PTSD is doing to his life?

The reason might be that he's getting a disability check each month as a result of his condition. His income is dependent on having PTSD, and if he recovers, his main source of livelihood might disappear with it.

Another reason might be that he was deeply wounded by a divorce many years ago. He lost his house and children in the process. He's fearful of getting into another romantic relationship that is likely to end badly. PTSD gives him a reason to not try.

These are obvious examples of secondary gain. When we work with participants in EFT workshops, we uncover a wide variety of subtle reasons that stand in the way of healing. One woman had been trying to lose weight for five years and had failed at every diet she tried. Her secondary gain turned out to be freedom from unwanted attention by men.

Another woman, this time with fibromyalgia, discovered that her secret benefit from the disease was that she didn't have to visit relatives she didn't like. She had a ready excuse for avoiding social obligations. She also got sympathetic attention from her husband and children for her suffering. If she gave up her painful disease, she might lose a degree of affection from her family and have to resume seeing the relatives she detested.

Just like Psychological Reversal, secondary gain prevents us from making progress on our healing journey. Correcting for these hidden obstacles to success is one of the first elements in EFTs Basic Recipe.

How EFT Corrects for Psychological Reversal

The first tapping point we use in the EFT routine is called the Karate Chop point, because it's located on the fleshy outer portion of the hand, the part used in karate to deliver a blow. EFT has you tap the Karate Chop point with the tips of the other four fingers of the opposite hand

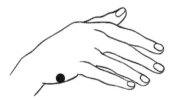

The Karate Chop (KC) Point

Repeat your affirmation emphatically three times while tapping your Karate Chop point. You've now corrected for psychological reversal, and set up your energy system for the next part of EFTs Basic Recipe, the Sequence.

The Sequence

You now tap on meridian end points in sequence. Tap firmly, but not harshly, with the tips of your first two fingers, about seven times on each point. The exact number is not important; it can be a few more or less than seven. You can tap on either the right or left side of your body, with either your dominant or nondominant hand.

First tap on the meridian endpoints found on the face. These are: (1) at the start of the eyebrow, where it joins the bridge of the nose; (2) on the outside edge of the eye socket; (3) on the bony ridge of the eye socket under the pupil; (4) under the nose; and (5) between the lower lip and the chin.

EB, SE, UE, UN and Ch Points

Then tap (6) on one of the collarbone points (see illustration). To locate this point, place a finger in the notch between your collarbones. Move your finger down about an inch and you'll feel a hollow in your breastbone.

Now move it to the side about an inch and you'll find a deep hollow below your collarbone. You've now located the collarbone acupressure point.

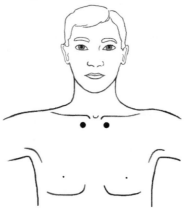

The Collarbone (CB) Points

About four inches below the armpit (for women, this is where a bra strap crosses), you'll find (7) the under the arm point.

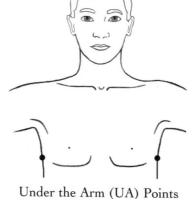

Under the Arm (UA) Points

The Reminder Phrase

Earlier, I emphasized the importance of exposure. Exposure therapy has been the subject of much research, which has shown that prolonged exposure to a problem, when coupled with techniques to calm the body, effectively treats traumatic stress. EFT incorporates exposure in the form of a Reminder Phrase. This is a brief phrase that keeps the problem at the front of your mind while you tap on the acupressure points. It keeps your energy system focused on the specific issue you're working on, rather than jumping to other thoughts and feelings. The aim of the Reminder Phrase is to bring the problem vividly into your experience, even though the emotionally triggering situation might not be present now.

For instance, if you have test anxiety, you use the Reminder Phrase to keep you focused on the fear, even though you aren't actually taking a test right now. That gives EFT an opportunity to shift the pattern in the absence of the real problem. You can also use EFT during an actual situation, such as when you're taking an actual test, but most of the time you're working on troublesome memories. The Reminder Phrase keeps you targeted on the problem. An example of a Reminder Phrase for test anxiety might be *"That test"* or *"The test I have to take tomorrow"* or *"That test I failed."* Other examples of Reminder Phrases are:

> *The beesting*
>
> *Dad hit me*
>
> *Friend doesn't respect me*

Lawyer's office

Sister told me I was fat

Car crash

This knee pain

Tap each point while repeating your Reminder Phrase. Then tune in to the problem again, and get a second SUD rating. The chances are good that your SUD score will now be much lower than it was before. These instructions might seem complicated the first time you read them, but you'll soon find you're able to complete a round of EFT tapping from memory in one to two minutes.

Let's now summarize the steps of EFTs Basic Recipe.

1. Assess your SUD level.

2. Insert the name of your problem into the Setup Statement: *"Even though I have (this problem), I deeply and completely accept myself."*

3. Tap continuously on the Karate Chop point while repeating the Setup Statement three times.

4. While repeating the Reminder Phrase, tap about seven times on the other seven points.

5. Test your results with a second SUD rating.

Isn't that simple? You now have a tool that, in just a minute or two, can effectively neutralize the emotional sting of old memories, as well as help you get through bad current situations. After a few rounds of tapping, you'll find you've effortlessly memorized the Basic Recipe, and you'll find yourself using it often in your daily life

If Your SUD Level Doesn't Come Down to 0

Sometimes a single round of tapping brings your SUD score to 0. Sometimes it only brings it down slightly. Your migraine might have been an 8, and after a round of EFT it's a 4. In these cases, we do EFT again. You can adjust your affirmation to acknowledge that a portion of the problem sill remains, for example, *"Even though I still have some of this migraine, I deeply and completely accept myself."* Hear are some further examples:

Even though I still feel some anger toward my friend for putting me down, I deeply and completely accept myself.

Even though I still have a little twinge of that knee pain, I deeply and completely accept myself.

Even though the beesting still smarts slightly, I deeply and completely accept myself.

Even though I'm still harboring some resentment toward my boss, I deeply and completely accept myself.

Even though I'm still somewhat frustrated with my daughter for breaking her agreement, I deeply and completely accept myself.

Even though I'm still upset when I think of being shipped to Iraq, I deeply and completely accept myself.

Adjust the Reminder Phrase accordingly, as in *"some anger still"* or *"remaining frustration"* or *"bit of pain"* or *"somewhat upset."*

EFT for You and Others

You can do EFT on yourself, as you've experienced during these practice rounds. You can also tap on others. Many therapists, life coaches, and other practitioners offer EFT professionally to clients. Personally I'm far more inclined to have clients tap on themselves during EFT sessions, even during the course of a therapy or coaching session. While the coach can tap on the client, having the client tap on themselves, along with some guidance by the coach, puts the power squarely in the hands of the client. The client is empowered by discovering that they are able to reduce their own emotional distress, and leaves the coaches office with a self-help tool at their fingertips any time they need it. In some jurisdictions, it is illegal or unethical for therapists to touch clients at all, and EFT when done only by the client is still effective in these cases.

The Importance of Targeting Specific Events

During EFT workshops, I sometimes write on the board:

The Three Most Important Things About EFT

Then, under that, I write:

Specific Events

Specific Events

Specific Events

It's my way of driving home the point that a focus on specific events is critical to success in EFT. In order to release old patterns of emotion and behavior, it's vital to identify and correct the specific events that gave rise to those problems. When you hear people say, "I tried EFT and it didn't work," the chances are good that they were tapping on generalities, instead of specifics.

An example of a generality is "self-esteem" or "depression" or "performance problems." These aren't specific events. Beneath these generalities is a collection of specific events. The person with low self-esteem might have been coloring a picture at the age of four when her mother walked in and criticized her for drawing outside the lines. She might have had another experience of a schoolteacher scolding her for playing with her hair during class in second grade, and a third experience of her first boyfriend deciding to ask another girl to the school dance. Together, those specific events contribute to the global pattern of low self-esteem. The way EFT works is that when the emotional trauma of those individual events is resolved, the whole pattern of low self-esteem can shift. If you tap on the big pattern, and omit the specific events, you're likely to have limited success.

When you think about how a big pattern like low self-esteem is established, this makes sense. It's built up out of many single events. Collectively, they form the whole pattern. The big pattern doesn't spring to life fully formed; it's built up gradually out of many similar experiences. The memories engraved in your brain are of individual events; one disappointing or traumatic memory at a time is encoded in your memory bank. When enough similar memories have accumulated, their commonalities combine to create a common theme like "poor self-esteem." Yet the theme originated as a series of specific events, and that's where EFT can be effectively applied.

You don't have to use EFT on every single event that contributed to the global theme. Usually, once a few of the most disturbing memories have lost their emotional impact, the whole pattern disappears. Memories that are similar lose their impact once the most vivid memories have been neutralized with EFT.

Tapping on global issues is the single most common mistake newcomers make with EFT. Using lists of tapping phrases from a website or a book, or tapping on generalities, is far less effective than tuning into the events that contributed to your global problem, and tapping on them. If you hear someone say, "EFT doesn't work," the chances are good they've been tapping globally rather than identifying specific events. Don't make this elementary mistake. List the events, one after the other, that stand out most vividly in your mind when you think about the global problem. Tap on each of them, and you'll usually find the global problem diminishing of its own accord. This is called the "generalization effect," and it's one of the key concepts in EFT.

Tapping on Aspects

EFT breaks traumatic events and other problems into smaller pieces called aspects. The reason for this is that the highest emotional charge is typically found in one small chunk of the event, rather than the entirety of the event. You might need to identify several different aspects, and tap on each of them, before the intensity of the whole event is reduced to a 0.

Here's an example of tapping on aspects, drawn from experience at an EFT workshop I taught. A woman in her late thirties volunteered as a subject. She'd had neck pain and limited range of motion since an automobile accident six years before. She could turn her head to the right most of the way but had only a few degrees of movement to the left. The accident had been a minor one, and why she still suffered six years later was something of a mystery to her.

I asked her to feel where in her body she felt the most intensity when recalling the accident, and she said it was in her upper chest. I then asked her about the first time she'd ever felt that way, and she said it was when she'd been involved in another auto accident at the age of eight. Her sister had been driving the car. We worked on each aspect of the early accident. The two girls had hit another car head on at low speed while driving around a bend on a country road. One emotionally triggering aspect was the moment she realized that a collision was unavoidable, and we tapped till that lost its force. We tapped on the sound of the crash, another aspect. She had been taken to a neighbor's house, bleeding from a cut on her head, and we tapped on that. We tapped on aspect after aspect. Still, her pain level didn't go down much, and her range of motion didn't improve.

Then she gasped and said, "I just remembered. My sister was only fifteen years old. She was underage. That day, I dared her to drive the family car, and we totaled it." Her guilt turned out to be the aspect that held the most emotional charge, and after we tapped on that, her pain disappeared, and she regained full range of motion in her neck. If we'd tapped on the later accident, or failed to uncover all the aspects, we might have thought, "EFT doesn't work."

Aspects can be pains, physical sensations, emotions, images, sounds, tastes, odors, fragments of an event, or beliefs. Make sure you dig deep for all the emotional charge held in each aspect of an event before you move on to the next one. One way of doing this is to check each sensory channel, and ask, "What did you hear/see/taste/touch/smell?" For one person, the burned-rubber smell of skidding tires might be the most terrifying aspect of a car accident. For another, it might be the smell of blood. Yet another person might remember most vividly the sound of the crash or the screams. For another person, the maximum emotional charge might be held in the feeling of terror at the moment of realization that the crash is inevitable. The pain itself might be an aspect. Guilt, or any other emotion, can be an aspect. For traumatic events, it's necessary to tap on each aspect.

Thorough exploration of all the aspects will usually yield a complete neutralization of the memory. If there's still some emotional charge left, the chances are good that you've missed an aspect, so go back and find out what shards of trauma might still be stuck in place.

Finding Core Issues

One of my favorite sayings during EFT workshops is "The problem is never the problem." What I mean by this is that the problem we complain about today usually bothers us only because it resembles an earlier problem. For example, if your spouse being late disturbs you, you may discover by digging deep with EFT that the real reason this behavior triggers you is that your mother didn't meet your needs in early childhood. Your spouse's behavior in the present day resembles, to your brain, the neglect you experienced in early childhood, so you react accordingly. You put a lot of energy into trying to change your spouse when the present-day person is not the source of the problem.

On the EFT Universe website, we have published hundreds of stories in which someone was no longer triggered by a present problem after the emotional charge was removed from a similar childhood event. Nothing changed in the present day, yet the very problem that so vexed a person before now carries zero emotional charge. That's the magic that happens once we neutralize core issues with EFT. Rather than being content with using EFT on surface problems, it's worth developing the skills to find and resolve the core issues that are at the root of the problem.

Here are some questions you might ask in order to identify core issues:

- Does the problem that's bothering you remind you of any events in your childhood? Tune into your body and feel your feelings. Then travel back in time to the first time in your life you ever felt that same sensation.

- What's the worst similar experience you ever had?

- If you were writing your autobiography, what chapter would you prefer to delete, as though it had never happened to you?

If you can't remember a specific childhood event, simply make up a fictional event in your mind. This kind of guessing usually turns out to be right on target. You're assembling the imagined event out of components of real events, and the imaginary event usually leads back to actual events you can tap on. Even if it doesn't, and you tap on the fictional event, you will usually experience an obvious release of tension.

The Generalization Effect

The *generalization effect* is a phenomenon you'll notice as you make progress with EFT. As you resolve the emotional sting of specific events, other events with a similar emotional signature also decrease in intensity. I once worked with a man at an EFT workshop whose father had beaten him many times during his childhood. His SUD level on the beatings was a 10. I asked him to recall the worst beating he'd ever suffered. He told me that when he was eight years old, his father had hit him so hard he had broken the boy's jaw. We tapped together on that terrible beating, and after working on all the aspects, his SUD dropped to a 0. I asked him for a SUD score on all the beatings, and his face softened. He said, "My dad got beat by his dad much worse than he beat me. My dad actually did a pretty good job considering how badly he was raised." My client's SUD level on all the beatings dropped considerably after we reduced the intensity of this one beating. That's an example of EFT's generalization effect. When you knock down an important domino, all the other dominos can fall.

This is very reassuring to clients who suffered from many instances of childhood abuse, the way my client at that workshop had suffered. You don't need to work through every single horrible incident. Often, simply collapsing the emotional intensity behind one incident is sufficient to collapse the intensity around similar incidents.

The reason our brains work this way is because of a group of neurons in the emotional center of the brain, the limbic system, called the hippocampus. The hippocampus has the job of comparing one event to the other. Suppose that, as a five-year-old child in Catholic school, you get beaten by a nun. Forty years later, you can't figure out why you feel uneasy around women wearing outfits that are black and white. The reason for your adult aversion to a black-and-white combination is that the hippocampus associates the colors of the nun's habit with the pain of the beating.

This was a brilliant evolutionary innovation for your ancestors. Perhaps these early humans were attacked by a tiger hiding in the long grass. The tiger's stripes mimicked the patterns of the grass yet there was something different there. Learning to spot a pattern, judge the differences, and react with fear saved your alert ancestors.

They gave birth to their children, who also learned, just a little bit better, how to respond to threats. After thousands of generations, you have a hippocampus at the center of your brain that is genetically engineered to evaluate every message flooding in from your senses, and pick out those associated with the possibility of danger. You see the woman wearing the black-and-white cocktail dress at a party, your hippocampus associates these colors with the nun who beat you, and you have an emotional response.

Yet the opposite is also true. Assume for a moment you're a man who is very shy when confronted with women at cocktail parties. He feels a rush of fear whenever he thinks about talking to an attractive woman dressed in black. He works with an EFT coach on his memories of getting beaten by the nun in Catholic school, and suddenly he finds himself able to talk easily to women at parties. Once the man's hippocampus breaks the connection between beatings and a black dress, it knows, for future reference, that the two phenomena are no longer connected.

This is the explanation the latest brain science gives us for the generalization effect. It's been noted in EFT for many years, and it's very comforting for those who've suffered many adverse experiences. You may need to tap on some of them, but you won't have to tap on all of them before the whole group is neutralized. Sometimes, like my client who was beaten repeatedly as a child, if you tap on a big one, the generalization effect reduces the emotional intensity of all similar experiences.

The Movie Technique and Tell the Story Technique

When you take an EFT workshop, the first key technique you learn is the Movie Technique. Why do we place such emphasis on the Movie Technique? The reason for this is that it combines many of the methods that are key to success with EFT.

The first thing the Movie Technique does is focus you on being specific. EFT is great at eliminating the emotional intensity you feel, as long as it's used on an actual concrete event ("John yelled at me in the meeting"), rather than a general statement ("My procrastination").

The Movie Technique has you identify a particular incident that has a big emotional charge for you, and systematically reduce that charge to 0. You picture the event in your mind's eye just as though it were a movie, and run through the movie scene by scene.

Whenever you reach a part of the movie that carries a big emotional charge, you stop and perform the EFT sequence. In this way, you reduce the intensity of each of the bad parts of the movie. EFT's related technique, Tell the Story, is done out loud, while the Movie Technique is typically done silently. You can use the Movie Technique with a client without them ever disclosing what the event was.

Try this with one of your own traumatic life events right now. Think of the event as though it were a scary movie. Make sure it's an event that lasts just a few minutes; if your movie lasts several hours or days, you've probably picked a general pattern. Try again, selecting a different event, till you have a movie that's just a few minutes long.

One example is a man whose general issue is "Distrust of Strangers." We trace it to a particular childhood incident that occurred when the man, whom we'll call John, was seven years old. His parents moved to a new town, and John found himself walking to a new school through a rough neighborhood. He encountered a group of bullies at school but always managed to avoid them. One day, walking back from school, he saw the bullies walking toward him. He crossed the street, hoping to avoid their attention. He wasn't successful, and he saw them point at him, then change course to intercept him. He knew he was due for a beating. They taunted him and shoved him, and he fell into the gutter. His mouth hit the pavement, and he chipped a tooth. Other kids gathered round and laughed at him, and the bullies moved off. He picked himself up and walked the rest of the way home.

If you were to apply EFT to John's general pattern, "Distrust of Strangers," you'd be tapping generally—and ineffectually. When instead you focus on the specific event, you're honing in on the life events that gave rise to the general pattern. A collection of events like John's beating can combine to create the general pattern.

Now give your movie a title. John might call his movie "The Bullies."

Start thinking about the movie at a point before the traumatic part began. For John, that would be when he was walking home from school, unaware of the events in store for him.

Now run your movie through your mind till the end. The end of the movie is usually a place where the bad events come to an end. For John, this might be when he picked himself up off the ground, and resumed his walk home.

Now let's add EFT to your movie. Here's the way you do this:

1. Think of the title of your movie. Rate your degree of your emotional distress around just the title, not the movie itself. For instance, on the distress scale of 0 to 10 where 0 is no distress and 10 represents maximum distress, you might be an 8 when you think of the title "The Meeting." Write down your movie title, and your number.

2. Work the movie title into an EFT Setup Statement. It might sound something like this: "Even though [Insert Your Movie Title Here], I deeply and completely accept myself." Then tap on the EFT acupressure points, while repeating the Setup Statement three times. Your distress level will typically go down. You may have to do EFT several times on the title for it to reach a low number like 0 or 1 or 2.

3. Once the title reaches a low number, think of the "neutral point" before the bad events in the movie began to take place. For John, the neutral point was when he was walking home from school, before the bullies saw him. Once you've identified the neutral point of your own movie, start running the movie through your mind, until you reach a point where the emotional intensity rises. In John's case,

the first emotionally intense point was when he saw the bullies.

4. Stop at this point, and assess your intensity number. It might have risen from a 1 to a 7, for instance. Then perform a round of EFT on that first emotional crescendo. For John, it might be, "Even though I saw the bullies turn toward me, I deeply and completely accept myself." Use the same kind of statement for your own problem: "Even though [first emotional crescendo], I deeply and completely accept myself." Keep tapping till your number drops to 0 or near 0, perhaps a 1 or 2.

5. Now rewind your mental movie to the neutral point, and start running it in your mind again. Stop at the first emotional crescendo. If you sail right through the first one you tapped on, you know you've really and truly resolved that aspect of the memory with EFT. Go on to the next crescendo. For John, this might have been when they shoved him into the gutter. When you've found your second emotional crescendo, then repeat the process. Assess your intensity number, do EFT, and keep tapping till your number is low. Even if your number is only a 3 or 4, stop and do EFT again. Don't push through low-intensity emotional crescendos; since you have the gift of freedom at your fingertips, use it on each part of the movie.

6. Rewind to the neutral point again, and repeat the process.

7. When you can replay the whole movie in your mind, from the neutral point, to the end of the movie when

your feelings are neutral again, you'll know you've resolved the whole event. You'll have dealt with all the aspects of the traumatic incident.

8. To truly test yourself, run through the movie, but exaggerate each sensory channel. Imagine the sights, sounds, smells, tastes, and other aspects of the movie as vividly as you possible can. If you've been running the movie silently in your mind, speak it out loud. When you cannot possibly make yourself upset, you're sure to have resolved the lingering emotional impact of the event. The effect is usually permanent.

When you work through enough individual movies in this way, the whole general pattern often vanishes. Perhaps John had forty events that contributed to his distrust of strangers. He might need to do the Movie Technique on all forty, but experience with EFT suggests that when you resolve just a few key events, perhaps five or ten of them, the rest fade in intensity, and the general pattern itself is neutralized.

The Tell the Story Technique is similar to the Movie Technique; usually the Movie Technique is performed silently while Tell the Story is out loud. One great benefit of the Movie Technique done silently is that the client does not have to disclose the nature of the problem. An event might be too triggering, or too embarrassing, or too emotionally overwhelming, to be spoken out loud. That's no problem with the Movie Technique, which allows EFT to work its magic without the necessity of disclosure on the part of the client. The privacy offered by the Movie Technique makes it very useful for clients who would rather not talk openly about troubling events.

Constricted Breathing

Here's a way to demonstrate how EFT can affect you physically. You can try this yourself right now. It's also often practiced as an onstage demonstration at EFT workshops. You simply take three deep breaths, stretching your lungs as far as they can expand. On the third breath, rate the extent of the expansion of your lungs on a 0 to 10 scale, with 0 being as constricted as possible, and 10 being as expanded as possible. Now perform several rounds of EFT using Setup Statements such as:

> *Even though my breathing is constricted...*
>
> *Even though my lungs will only expand to an 8...*
>
> *Even though I have this physical problem that prevents me breathing deeply...*

Now take another deep breath and rate your level of expansion. Usually there's substantial improvement. Now focus on any emotional contributors to constricted breathing. Use questions like:

> *What life events can I associate with breathing problems?*
>
> *Are there places in my life where I feel restricted?*
>
> *If I simply guess at an emotional reason for my constricted breathing, what might it be?*

Now tap on any issues surfaced by these questions. After your intensity is reduced, take another deep breath and rate how far your lungs are now expanding. Even if you were a 10 earlier, you might now find you're an 11 or 14.

The Personal Peace Procedure

The Personal Peace Procedure consists of listing every specific troublesome event in your life and systematically using EFT to tap away the emotional impact of these events. With due diligence, you knock over every negative domino on your emotional playing board and, in so doing, remove significant sources of both emotional and physical ailments. You experience personal peace, which improves your work and home relationships, your health, and every other area of your life.

Tapping on large numbers of events one by one might seem like a daunting task, but we'll show you in the next few paragraphs how you can accomplish it quickly and efficiently. Because of EFT's generalization effect, where tapping on one issue reduces the intensity of similar issues, you'll typically find the process going much faster than you imagined.

Removing the emotional charge from your specific events results in less and less internal conflict. Less internal conflict results, in turn, in greater personal peace and less suffering on all levels—physical, mental, emotional, and spiritual. For many people, the Personal Peace Procedure has led to the complete cessation of lifelong issues that other methods did not resolve. You'll find stories on the EFT Universe website written by people who describe relief from physical maladies like headaches, breathing difficulties, and digestive disorders. You'll read other stories of people who used EFT to help them deal with the stress associated with AIDS, multiple sclerosis, and cancer. Unresolved anger, traumas, guilt, or grief contributes to physical illness, and cannot be medicated away. EFT addresses these emotional contributors to physical disease.

Here's how to do the Personal Peace Procedure:

1. List every specific troublesome event in your life that you can remember. Write them down in a Personal Peace Procedure journal. "Troublesome" means it caused you some form of discomfort. If you listed fewer than fifty events, try harder to remember more. Many people find hundreds. Some bad events you recall may not seem to cause you any current discomfort. List them anyway. The fact that they came to mind suggests they may need resolution. As you list them, give each specific event a title, like it's a short movie, such as: Mom slapped me that time in the car; I stole my brother's baseball cap; I slipped and fell in front of everybody at the ice skating rink; My third grade class ridiculed me when I gave that speech; Dad locked me in the toolshed overnight; Mrs. Simmons told me I was dumb.

2. When your list is finished, choose the biggest dominoes on your board, that is, the events that have the most emotional charge for you. Apply EFT to them,

one at a time, until the SUD level for each event is 0. You might find yourself laughing about an event that used to bring you to tears; you might find a memory fading. Pay attention to any aspects that arise and treat them as separate dominoes, by tapping for each aspect separately. Make sure you tap on each event until it is resolved. If you find yourself unable to rate the intensity of a bad event on the 0-10 scale, you might be dissociating, or repressing a memory. One solution to this problem is to tap ten rounds of EFT on every aspect of the event you are able to recall. You might then find the event emerging into clearer focus but without the same high degree of emotional charge.

3. After you have removed the biggest dominoes, pick the next biggest, and work on down the line.

4. If you can, clear at least one of your specific events, preferably three, daily for three months. By taking only minutes per day, in three months you will have cleared 90 to 270 specific events. You will likely discover that your body feels better, that your threshold for getting upset is much lower, your relationships have improved, and many of your old issues have disappeared. If you revisit specific events you wrote down in your Personal Peace Procedure journal, you will likely discover that the former intensity has evaporated. Pay attention to improvements in your blood pressure, pulse, and respiratory capacity. EFT often produces subtle but measurable changes

in your health, and you may miss them if you aren't looking for them.

5. After knocking down all your dominoes, you may feel so much better that you're tempted to alter the dosages of medications your doctor has prescribed. Never make any such changes without consulting with your physician. Your doctor is your partner in your healing journey. Tell your doctor that you're working on your emotional issues with EFT, since most health-care professionals are acutely aware of the contribution that stress makes to disease.

The Personal Peace Procedure does not take the place of EFT training, nor does it take the place of assistance from a qualified EFT practitioner. It is an excellent supplement to EFT workshops and help from EFT practitioners. EFT's full range of resources is designed to work effectively together for the best healing results.

Is It Working Yet?

Sometimes EFT's benefits are blindingly obvious. In the introductory video on the home page of the EFT Universe website, you see a TV reporter with a lifelong fear of spiders receiving a tapping session. Afterward, in a dramatic turnaround, she's able to stroke a giant hairy tarantula spider she's holding in the palm of her hand.

Other times, EFTs effects are subtler and you have to pay close attention to spot them. A friend of mine who has had a lifelong fear of driving in high-speed traffic remarked to me recently that her old fear is completely gone. Over the past year, each time she felt anxious about driving, she pulled her car to the side of the road and tapped. It took many trips and much tapping, but subtle changes gradually took effect. Thanks to EFT she has emotional freedom and drives without fear. She also has another great benefit, in the form of a closer bond to her daughter and baby granddaughter. They live two hours drive away and, previously, her dread of traffic kept her from visiting them. Now she's able to make the drive with joyful anticipation of playing with her granddaughter.

If you seem not to be making progress on a particular problem despite using EFT, look for other positive changes that might be happening in your life. Stress affects every system in the body, and once you relieve it with EFT, you might find improvements in unexpected areas. For instance, when stressed, the capillaries in your digestive system constrict, impeding digestion. Many people with digestive problems report improvement after EFT. Stress also redistributes biological resources away from your reproductive system. You'll find many stories on EFT Universe of people whose sex lives improved dramatically as a by-product of healing emotional issues. Stress affects your muscular and circulatory systems; many people report that muscular aches and pains disappear after EFT, and their blood circulation improves. Just as stress is pervasive, relaxation is pervasive, and when we release our emotional bonds with EFT, the relaxing effects are felt all over the body. So perhaps your sore knee has only improved slightly, but you're sleeping better, having fewer respiratory problems, and getting along better with your coworkers.

Saying the Right Words

A common misconception is that you have to say just the right words while tapping in order for EFT to be effective. The truth is that focusing on the problem is more important than the exact words you're using. It's the exposure to the troubling issue that directs healing energy to the right place; the words are just a guide.

Many practitioners write down tapping scripts with lists of affirmations you can use. These can be useful. However, your own words are usually able to capture the full intensity of your emotions in a way that is not possible using other people's words. The way you form language is associated with the configuration of the neural network in your brain. You want the neural pathways along which stress signals travel to be very active while you tap. Using your own words is more likely to awaken that neural pathway fully than using even the most eloquent words suggested by someone else. By all means use tapping scripts if they're available, to nudge you in the right direction. At the same time, utilize the power of prolonged exposure by focusing your mind completely on your own experience. Your mind and body have a healing wisdom that usually directs healing power toward the place where it is most urgently required.

The Next Steps on Your EFT Journey

Now that you've entered the world of EFT, you'll find it to be a rich and supportive place. On the EFT Universe website, you'll find stories written by thousands of people, from all over the world, describing success with an enormous variety of problems. Locate success stories on your particular problem by using the site's drop-down menu, which lists issues alphabetically: Addictions, ADHD, Anxiety, Depression, and so on. Read these stories for insights on how to apply EFT to your particular case. They'll inspire you in your quest for full healing.

Our certified practitioners are a wonderful resource. They've gone through rigorous training in Clinical EFT and have honed their skills with many clients. Many of them work via telephone or videoconferencing, so if you don't find the perfect practitioner in your geographic area, you can still get expert help with remote sessions. While EFT is primarily a self-help tool and you can get great results alone, you'll find the insight that comes from an outside observer can often alert you to behavior patterns and solutions you can't find by yourself.

Take an EFT workshop. EFT Universe offers more than a hundred workshops each year, all over the world, and you're likely to find a Level 1 and 2 workshop close to you. You'll make friends, see expert demonstrations, and learn EFT systematically. Each workshop contains eight learning modules, and each module builds on the one before. Fifteen years' experience in training thousands of people in EFT has shown us exactly how people learn EFT competently and quickly, and provided the background knowledge to design these trainings. Read the many testimonials on the website to see how deeply transformational the EFT workshops are.

The EFT Universe newsletter is the medium that keeps the whole EFT world connected. Read the stories published there weekly to stay inspired and to learn about new uses for EFT. Write your own experiences and submit them to the newsletter. Post comments on the EFT Universe Facebook page, and comment in the blogs.

If you'd like to help others access the benefits you have gained from EFT, you might consider volunteering your services. There are dozens of ways to support EFT's growth and progress. You can join a tapping circle, or start one yourself. You can donate to EFT research and humanitarian efforts. You can offer tapping sessions to people who are suffering through one of EFT's humanitarian projects, like those that have reached thousands in Haiti, Rwanda, and elsewhere. You can let your friends know about EFT.

EFT has reached millions of people worldwide with its healing magic but is still in its infancy. By reading this book and practicing this work, you're joining a healing revolution that has the potential to radically reduce human suffering. Imagine if the benefits you've already experienced could be shared by every child, every sick person, every anxious or stressed person in the world. The trajectory of human history would be very different. I'm committed to helping create this shift however I can, and I invite you to join me and all the other people of goodwill in making this vision of a transformed future a reality.

2

Tapping Away Cravings

Your First Experience of Tapping for Cravings

Imagine gathering up a big bowl of your favorite chocolate. Piece by piece, you add it to the bowl. Then imagine yourself walking over to the trash can and throwing the whole bowl away.

Do you have an emotional reaction in your body when I describe that scene? That's not unusual, because most of us have a hard time throwing food away, but imagining throwing away a food you crave can elicit the strongest possible reactions. Picture the scene again. Imagine selecting those pieces of chocolate, then throwing the whole bowl away. Assess your level of emotional triggering, with 10 being maximum and 0 being minimum. Then tap and do EFT several times while picturing the chocolate going into the trash. The chances are good that your number will drop way down.

Throwing chocolate into the trash is something I do on a regular basis. On the second day of every Level 1 workshop, we offer a cravings exercise, and we bring chocolate into the room to allow workshop participants to experience their cravings. Most of them have a high number, with many at a 10.

What's astonishing is to see what happens next. Sure, EFT brings their numbers way down. Studies show the average drop in cravings is 83 percent after about thirty minutes of tapping on emotional events in their lives (Church & Brooks, 2010).

That's the last module of the workshop, and participants leave afterward. They gather their belongings, chat, make friends, and leave the room. The chocolate we used to test their cravings lies forgotten, strewn all over the tables. They get up and walk away, with no more thought given to the chocolate than to the empty coffee cups and water bottles in the room.

When I and the other workshop staff clean up, we then throw all that chocolate in the trash, because no-one wants it. In the course of my teaching career, I've probably thrown hundreds of pounds of chocolate into the trash after EFT Level 1 workshops!

Using EFT to reduce cravings gives you great leverage during a weight loss program. You can tap directly on your cravings, and also tap on specific emotional events associated with the item you crave. When cravings are high, your SUD numbers are high, and you have full access to the experience of craving. Periods of peak intensity bring the issue to the forefront of your awareness, and that's the perfect time to tap.

A craving is a strong desire, an intense longing, for a special something. It can be for anything, even raw carrots, but among those who would like to lose weight, raw carrot cravings are rare. Ice cream, chocolate, macaroni and cheese, pound cake, cookies, and other filling, satisfying, high-fat, high-carb treats are the comfort foods that keep calling.

You might find it hard to believe that EFT can take away your craving for a food you find irresistible. So let's try it in practice. Grab the food you crave most right now. Look at the food. Rate your intensity of longing on a scale from 0 to 10, and write down your number here: SUD before: _____. Then, tap on your Karate Chop point continuously while saying this Setup Statement out loud three times:

> *Even though I have this incredible craving for _____, I deeply and completely accept myself.*

Now tap through all the points from top to bottom while using the name of the food as your Reminder Phrase. After you get to the last point, rate your level of craving a second time: SUD after: _____. You'll probably find that your number has gone down quite a bit. In live workshops, or Skinny Genes coaching calls, I find that most people's SUD goes down by at least two points. A few people in the group are startled to find that their craving level has dropped to a 0. Congratulations! You've now had your first experience of using EFT for cravings. It's that simple to get started, and you'll unlock more and more of the power of EFT as you continue to use it.

If the simple Setup you just used doesn't do the trick, enhancing the description usually will. Try smelling the item, tasting just a little, holding it in you hand, or doing anything else that might help you discover apsects of your craving that haven't been addressed yet, and incorporate these observations into your Setup. For example:

Even though that chocolate is making my mouth water and I can't even look at it without drooling, I deeply and completely accept myself.

Even though I really want those potato chips, and I can already smell how fresh and crispy they would be if I were to open that bag, I deeply and completely accept myself.

Once their cravings have been "tapped away," people often find it difficult to taste, touch, or even look at the very same foods they were excited about moments before. Someone who loves potato chips will frown and say, "The whole package smells rancid." A chocolate lover will complain that a fresh, expensive piece tastes weird or waxy.

To appreciate how quickly and effectively EFT can work for your own issues, including weight loss and uncontrollable cravings, consider the following reports.

Linda Compton started a "Roots of Weight" class and used EFT to help with the many addictive substances that contribute to being overweight. I think you will find her message filled with evidence about how EFT works in this area. Some people seemingly get completely over their cravings rapidly while others have increased cravings for something else.

Intense Cravings in a Weight-loss Class

by Linda Compton

At one point, I started a class for women called the Roots of Weight. There were ten women in the class and we met every Thursday from 7 to 9 p.m.

At the third class I taught EFT and the women tapped for everything from chips to cigarettes, Milano cookies, StarBucks peanut butter cookies, wine, and vodka.

One woman said she had the unusual habit of chewing eight packs of gum every night. She would fall asleep chewing gum, wake up two hours later, and eat a one-pound pack of raisins. Then she would chew more gum and fall asleep. The gum had to come from a particular store and it had to be Doublemint in the green wrapper and Spearmint in the white wrapper. She would repeat this cycle every night.

She told me, "I have a master's degree in psychology. I should be able to stop this, but I feel out of control."

She tapped for the raisins only and ten days later, she still doesn't want them. She told me she looked at the raisins on the shelf and thought, "Oh, there are those raisins." She had no desire to eat the raisins. She didn't crave them any more at all. And although she was happy about the raisins, she said the intensity of the craving for the gum increased. Next, she tapped for the gum chewing. She called a few days later to say that she had not had any gum, nor did she want any. She had four packs in her drawer and had absolutely no craving for it.

I spoke with her shortly thereafter and she said this is a miracle. She has been doing this behavior of chewing gum and eating raisins all night for two years. She made numerous visits to the doctor and was told not to worry about it, that it would soon pass. She even brought up the idea that she might have a nutritional deficiency, like a lack of chromium, but the doctor told her the research wasn't in on that. She is ecstatic.

She is not the only one in the class who stopped cravings. Another woman eats five small donuts a day. She is down to one and a half. Another ate three bags of corn nuts last Wednesday and is addicted to potato chips, pork rinds, and anything salty. She told me she hasn't had any of those items since she tapped for her cravings.

I tapped for sugar with the class and haven't had any since. I have also let go of coffee, popcorn, and ice cream. And although we could be tapping for all these food items at one time, I know that particular cravings are motivated by particular emotions and sometimes physical conditions.

One friend let go of the grief she had been feeling for her deceased mother. There were songs she could not stand to listen to and is now okay with. Another client let go of coffee and her fear of selling real estate. She now is working full time selling real estate and teases me about "f-ing up her coffee thing."

In my Roots of Weight class, these women are exploring the deep roots of their beliefs so that they can see clearly how the beliefs branch out to undesired behaviors, creating undesired results, such as undesired weight. One of the women found this so profound that she downloaded *The EFT Manual* to study.

This is so wonderful. The woman with the gum-chewing habit demonstrates how large this whole energy psychology is. She just can't believe she only had to tap once to heal it.

❋ ❋ ❋

Whether it is chocolate, popcorn, or a special snack or dessert, our systems can develop a major case of the Yum-Yums and cause us to overeat many things. Collette Streicher's client faced this dilemma with regard to peanuts and used EFT to effectively diminish her cravings.

Notice how Colette's client started with a craving, peeled away emotional layers, and uncovered a supporting emotional issue. It's the underlying issues we really want to address, so whenever you're tapping, be on the lookout for them.

Overcoming a Food Craving
by Collette Streicher and Chris

My client, Chris, sent me this great letter about how she eliminated a peanut craving with all the details and some humor, too. She hopes it can help others.

Dear Colette,

I am writing this note to tell you how much the EFT has been helping me with food cravings. What I absolutely love about working with this tool is the flexibility and availability of using my fingertips to conquer problems that used to overwhelm me.

I have long struggled with food issues. I know I have a lot of great reasons to lose weight, but I could never get past the thought that I would have to let go of food that I really loved, especially peanuts. If I were ever stranded on a desert island, it would be a long, long time before I starved because you can bet I would have a huge pack of peanuts in my purse, one in a certain pocket of my briefcase, and if I had driven to that island, there would be a jar or two rolling around on the car's floorboard. So, as I've learned, from you and others on the EFT website, I started with whatever feeling came up first.

Even though I really can't stand the idea of giving up peanuts, I deeply and completely accept myself.

Even though I'm angry that I am forced to give up peanuts…

Forced? Who was forcing me? I couldn't think of anyone standing between peanuts and me. So I went with that.

Even though I don't know who is forcing me to stop eating peanuts…

Even though it is me who is being so forceful…

Even though I feel forceful when I am eating peanuts...

Now this rang true for me. I have always known that part of the appeal of nuts for me is the physical crunching and chewing. I guess I feel like I am getting somewhere by doing all that chewing.

Even though chewing and crunching feels forceful...

Then as I was tapping the above statement, it came to me. I used to get angry at my ex-husband, the one who was constantly nagging me about losing weight.

Even though my ex tried to force me to lose weight, I ate anyway, 'cause nobody can stop me if I don't want to stop.

Even though I can't say anything about not wanting to lose weight, I can chew and chew these peanuts forcefully.

Then I really got it that the act of chewing was about biting back my feelings and biting back my words. I could feel the anger in my jaws! By this time I was just tapping on the points with these Reminder Phrases:

This biting back my feelings.

This biting back my words.

These angry jaws.

These forceful jaws.

Then I felt sad because that was the only way I could express myself in that situation, so again, I tapped on:

This sadness.

This peanut sadness.

This chewing sadness.

This feeling alone.

Then I felt better, so I stopped. Most of the anger was gone. I didn't test myself, because I was a little melancholy that I had to do all this work around peanuts and chewing. I could have tapped on the shame of having this issue in the first place, but I didn't. I know if I had been in a session with you, we might have gone deeper, but I felt satisfied at the time. In fact, I didn't really think to see if peanuts still had a charge with me. I started doing something else.

The oddest thing (though maybe not to you) was that I didn't even think about peanuts again until I was in line at the bank and I saw the emergency package I kept in my purse. I hadn't eaten peanuts in days! Then it became weeks. I can truthfully say I am not peanutty anymore!

Notice Chris's references to anger, sadness, shame, and feeling alone. These are all aspects of the issue with her ex-husband. If the peanut craving came back after this session, or if the overall food issue persisted, I might look deeper into the specific events with her ex-husband, or see if there is something similar in childhood to address.

❊ ❊ ❊

Alyson Raworth's client in Scotland had a major chocolate craving. Notice how she amplifies the "yumminess" and appeal of the chocolate to truly tune her client into the craving. Nestlé's Yorkies, which are popular in the U.K., are marketed as a man's chocolate bar. In this session, Alyson has her client massage his Sore Spot on the upper chest instead of tapping the Karate Chop point while reciting his Setup Phrase. The two can be used interchangeably. For more about the Sore Spot, see Appendix A.

Hitting a Chocolate Craving Head-on

by Alyson Raworth

I have been doing sessions with a male client who desperately wanted to lose weight but who had a chocolate fixation. He tried and tried but although he seemed to have willpower, he didn't have enough for this chocolate thing.

As the rest of his diet was sensible, I concentrated on the chocolate. I put some pieces of Yorkie on the table in front of him. His level of desire was above a 10.

I started with having him massage his Sore Spot while saying:

Even though my chocolate thing is intense, I love my body. Although I really love and want that yummy Yorkie, I love and respect my body.

His level went down to 9.

Then I did a big one:

Even though I can taste the texture of that gorgeous velvety sweetness which is just so yummy that my tongue is swirling round in my mouth in anticipation of popping that piece in front of me into my mouth, I love and respect myself and choose to have the imagination to see myself slim.

He looked strangely at me and had one of those sighs. He said that he had never been able to imagine himself actually slim!

The wording was then changed to:

Even though I am just an old tub of lard, not good for anything, not even good for getting slim, I do love and respect my body and mind.

He laughed and laughed at that and said that the chocolate looked different now. I asked him to explain and he said that it had somehow lost its appeal!

That was the turning point. I asked him how much he wanted to eat the chocolate now and he said that he didn't want it at all. His level was a complete 0! Brilliant!

We are going to work on his self-image next and build up confidence and self-esteem.

* * *

You may have noticed the use of "I love and respect my body" in the preceding report's Setup Phrases. That statement is a cousin to "I deeply and completely accept myself" because it adds an element of self-acceptance to the Setup.

You may have also noticed "I choose to have the imagination to see myself slim." This is an EFT variation that uses affirmations to trigger new aspects. Obviously, Alyson was savvy enough to know that an overall self-image issue might have been a bigger contributor to the craving than the Yorkie. By using the affirmation, she was able to test the waters and found a valuable direction for her next round of tapping.

If a craving doesn't disappear in record time, it is probably attached to an emotional issue that needs to be addressed before the craving can be diminished. Sergio Lizarraga from Mexico illustrates this next with a brief report.

Chocolate Cravings and Childhood Poverty
by Sergio Lizarraga

A friend was struggling with her weight issues. I introduced her to a basic routine of EFT to help eliminate her chocolate cravings, which were the major contributor to her overweight problem. But when she tapped for her chocolate cravings directly, it did not help at all. When we talked about it later on, she told me about her childhood in poverty and how she could not have candies or chocolates then. Now that she is an adult she wants the chocolates she could not have as a child. I suggested tapping on:

Even though I could not have chocolate when I was a child, I deeply and completely accept myself.

Even though I wanted a chocolate when I was a child...

Three weeks later she contacted me again, very happy. She says that by doing the tapping in this way her craving totally disappeared. Now she is losing weight and feeling much better. Needless to say she is using EFT for a lot of issues in her life and for her family as well.

Something interesting to mention here is that I have never met my friend in person. We got in touch through a Spanish EFT webpage that I own. All the conversations and ideas shared have been done through instant messages and emails!

※ ※ ※

In the preceding case, Sergio was able to find some underlying emotional issues connected to the craving and apparently didn't have to go any further. When using EFT for your own craving, if you have tapped on similar issues and still aren't seeing results, you could be more specific by working with the events themselves, like "the time when my father wouldn't let me have chocolate..." and any others that cause intensity. Once all the related memories have lost their "grip," that part of the issue is likely to be released for good.

In this next article by Dr. Shelley Malka, you will see how she helped her client get to the true emotional issues behind cravings that just wouldn't go away. Notice how the tapping process and Shelley's gentle suggestions along the way reduced a frustrating craving down to what seems to be a specific event. Also note how Shelley was able to address the event even though she didn't know any of the details. This case illustrates why it is often important to seek the help of an experienced professional for best results.

What was *Really* Behind Those Cravings?

by Dr. Shelley Malka

The following story demonstrates clearly that any craving or addiction is not about the object we crave at all. Rather, the craved object is a substitute for anxiety that lies beneath the addiction. Once we access that disallowed or forbidden feeling, the craving disappears as if by magic. And you as the therapist or helper don't have to know what's really going on for this process to work wonders.

Odette was a client I knew well. She called me over the phone one day asking me to please help her work through her craving for chocolate and cake that had been with her the last few days. Intensity for these foods was building and she knew she couldn't hold out much longer on her own without blowing her diet. She had tapped consistently but couldn't get to whatever it was that was clearly holding up her craving.

"What triggered this?" I asked. "You've been much better with chocolate and cake recently."

"I know I have," she said. "That's why I'm so frustrated. I just can't work this one out and the craving is ballooning."

"Okay," I said. "Just go to the Karate Chop point and let's start."

Even though I don't know what triggered this... I was doing fine...doing much better...and then the last few days I haven't been able to get cake out of my mind...and chocolate...I don't know why...

Nothing emerged and, looking for a door to go in, I asked if she had a craving right then. She said, "No, not right now, but I know that if I wasn't on the phone to you, I'd head straight for the chocolate."

"You don't have the craving now perhaps because I'm here and you feel safe." I let her tap on this awareness a bit. "When did you have this craving? Could you allow your inner mind to go to where you were, what was happening when you first noticed this feeling of needing cake?" Tap, tap.

"Well I think the first time I started this cake-feeling I was in the car. If there'd been a place to buy chocolate, I think I would have stopped right there."

"Go into that moment," I suggested "Just be in the car and allow that feeling to surface...I'm in the car...just tap around the points in the car and all of a sudden I want cake...all of a sudden I'm looking around for somewhere to buy chocolate." Her level of intensity was between 5 and 6 on a scale of 0 to 10.

Even though I'm a 5 or 6 right now...And I don't know what it is...Even though it's intensifying, that's good, that's why I phoned you, to find out what this is...

At that moment, she burst out crying. "I think I do know," she said. "I can't believe it's this…I had no idea. I can't believe it's this…but that's what's coming up."

We tapped a few rounds on "this awareness… this realization." Then she said, "And it's a lose-lose situation!" I immediately referred her back to the Karate Chop point.

Even though it's a lose-lose situation…

Even though no matter what I do, I'll lose out…

We did quite a bit of this. I didn't add anything. I wanted whatever needed to surface, to just float up to consciousness. We tapped on the feelings that arose.

Even though I'm scared…

Whenever there's a fear we're afraid to face—fear of the fear as it's often called—we're usually holding an underlying belief that if we know what that fear is, we won't be able to cope with it. So I threw this in:

Even though I'm scared, and I don't know if I can handle it…And that's making me crave chocolate and cake…

"That's right!" she exclaimed. "I don't!" More sobs. I backtracked here so she could process the steps and integrate the parts as we traveled round and round the points:

It's a lose-lose situation and I'm scared because I don't know if I can handle it…no matter what I do, I'll lose and I don't know if I can handle that…it's mak-

ing me crave chocolate and cake because I'm so anxious about this lose-lose…I want to stuff it down with chocolate and cake.

"Anything!" she cried. "Even chicken and potatoes!" Well, this was a new aspect she hadn't realized before, so I took her back to the Karate Chop point:

Even though this lose-lose is making me crave anything, even chicken and potatoes, and it's all to keep my anxiety down…

This anxiety that I can't handle the lose-lose…this anxiety that I can't handle my feelings about this lose-lose…calming this anxiety with any food so that I can obsess about food and my weight rather than deal with this lose-lose anxiety.

"Yeah," she agreed, "that's what I do, all right." But she was definitely calmer, having found the issue underpinning her craving.

We checked her craving. She was still a 4 or 5 on the 0-to-10 scale, even though she had stopped crying. "It's because I haven't found the core yet," she said. "And I'm anxious about not finding it."

We did a whole lot more tapping on this—to calm her, to make her anxiety okay, to challenge the assumptions in her unconscious mind that she couldn't handle the lose-lose (whatever that was, since I had no clue). I asked what the craving was like and she said it was still 4 or 5 out of 10 "because I don't know how he'll take it." Here was another aspect that slipped out, so seemingly innocuous as to have us believe she'd known about it all along.

Even though I don't know how he'll take it…

Her tears and sobs started up again.

Even though I have no idea how he'll take it and that's the real concern, the real anxiety…up to now I haven't allowed myself to know how anxious I am about that…I was scared I wouldn't be able to handle it…I truly was scared to know this because it seemed too big for me…

By now her voice was softer and more pliable. Things had changed. So we checked her craving again. "It's much better!" she said. "I don't need the chocolate anymore!"

I asked her to do what she could to get that craving back either for chocolate, or cake or chicken and potatoes or anything I got her to make the images bigger and brighter and smell the chocolate in her mind… but the craving was gone. Furthermore, Odette not only knew she could now handle her feelings about how he'd take it but it was also no longer lose-lose. She had found a solution to make it easy.

I said, "So now that you know what IT is, you can tap for that, without me, and you no longer have to eat yourself into oblivion." She laughed again. "I feel such relief. It always amazes me how it's never about the cake or the chocolate, is it?" I said goodbye to Odette and looked at my watch. The entire session had taken approximately fifteen minutes. And I never did find out what "it" was.

✳ ✳ ✳

EFT usually gets rid of immediate cravings in short order. When that doesn't happen, there is almost always a deeper issue behind the craving. Such was the case in this article by Ilana Weiler from Israel. Note how important memories showed up during the EFT process, pointing the way to the problem's core issue.

A Craving Vanishes for a Skeptical Doctor

by Ilana Weiler

Recently I attended a birthday party and had the pleasure of meeting a group of amazing women. I assume we all know that scenario where we find ourselves in a social gathering and sooner or later the subject of EFT is brought up. One of the women said, "What is this EFT? Is it this stupid thing where one taps on himself looking like a monkey?"

Well, that's a chance to catch the ball. She is a highly positioned doctor but, nonetheless, I asked her if she would like to try it. To my great surprise, she agreed. I am writing all the details of this event to encourage you, the reader who doesn't yet feel confident with EFT, to not only Try It on Everything but also Try It on Everybody—anytime.

So this woman (I will call her Lea), wanted to try EFT for her uncontrollable desire for sweets. I asked her what on the table she wanted to eat the most. She said she wanted everything, but mostly the cake. On the scale of 0 to 10 she wanted it at a level of 8. I asked her what it was about that cake that she wanted so much. She said it was the sweetness of it.

Even though I want that sweet cake so much...

We used the words sweet, sweet cake, and sweetness as Reminder Phrases.

After one round Lea said, "I am like an elephant that grabs everything sweet with its trunk. I am like a vacuum cleaner."

After a few rounds I handed her the piece of cake. Now it had a level of intensity of 6 out of 10. We kept tapping while she suddenly said, "Oh, I have a flashback of a memory when I was about three years old. My father used to buy me those sugar candies that looked like crystals."

I kept tapping on her as she talked, astonished by the fact she had recalled a memory she had never remembered in fifty years. And then came another. She said, "I remember we used to go to the zoo, and my father always had these little bags filled with sweets. And now I remember how he used to feed me patiently this sweet porridge."

She was absolutely a pleasure to work with, so freely cooperating with the process of EFT. I was very touched by this gush of memories and she was, too. I asked Lea if she missed her father and she said she missed him terribly. Bingo.

Even though I miss my father terribly...physically and emotionally I miss my father...I miss him so much.

Even though I miss my sweet father, I miss our sweet relationship, I miss all those sweet memories, I accept my feelings and respect myself.

For Reminder Phrases, we used *my sweet father... our sweet relationship...my sweet memories.*

She said she understood that this craving for sugar was a substitute for her relationship with her father. I continually tapped on her as she suddenly said she could see herself as an adolescent, wearing a medallion of the peace symbol. "I want to make peace within me," she said.

After tapping for that I gave her the piece of cake and she repelled it with her whole body. "I can't even think of putting it in my mouth!" It was an amazing demonstration of getting to the core issue quickly. The whole thing took about twenty minutes. What a sweet process!

❀ ❀ ❀

In the next report, Dorothy Goudie from New Zealand gives us a classic example of how EFT neutralized a craving for ice cream. Notice the specific language she and her client used to describe the craving. If you just try to describe your craving the way you would to a good friend, this is the kind of language you might use. These detailed descriptions in the Setup help trigger the intensity more completely, and they assist the tapping process in correcting the related disruptions.

EFT for Ice Cream Cravings

by Dorothy Goudie

A woman with a weight problem narrowed her cravings down to several items with one being over-indulgence in ice cream—especially the ones coated in chocolate.

In New Zealand we have a chocolate-coated ice cream on a stick called a Topsy. This was her favorite. As we talked about the Topsy, she rated her craving at an intensity level of 10 out of 10. When I produced one and started to peel the wrapper off, she was salivating. By the time I put it in her hand and asked her just to smell it, her craving was way over a 10.

We put the ice cream to one side, away from her but where she could see it. While tapping on her Karate Chop point, I started by saying, *"I just love those Topsys."*

"Oh!" she exclaimed, "I can smell that beautiful sweet smell on your fingers." At this point she took over with the words pouring out, so I just repeated back to her what she was saying and continuously tapped while she was doing this.

The smell in particular is divine, and the creamy feel of the chocolate with the cool ice cream just melts in your mouth and flows over your tongue.

I just love ice cream, it is sooo good, and I can't get enough of it.

Love the taste, love the smell, just love everything about ice cream.

Surely ice cream can't be that fattening.

Oh I know it is but I just can't resist, love that cool feel in the mouth.

Love that smell, it's so sweet.

Delicious, makes me feel so good.

We did six or seven rounds of tapping on this and then took a pause while I asked how she was feeling now about ice cream. She had a blank look on her face, quite startled. It was almost as though it took a moment or two to realize that her previous thoughts were no longer so.

I suggested that she take another smell of the Topsy and give me a rating on the 0-to-10 scale. She took the ice cream and sniffed, and sniffed again, and with shock on her face said, "I can't smell anything. It's like plastic. My nose must be blocked. Did you switch the ice cream? You couldn't have done that, I was watching. I don't want to eat that. There is no pleasure in something that smells like plastic."

I suggested that she might like to take a bite of it and test it but she refused, saying that she couldn't bear to eat something that smelled like that.

An hour later, as she was ready to leave, we tested again with the same results. The intensity of her craving was still at a 0. She could not believe that her lifetime passion for ice cream could vanish in ten minutes.

I then asked her to take the Topsy and throw it in the rubbish. She took the ice cream in her hand and just stopped, shock showing in her face and body. She said, "I can't throw this away, what a waste, you could wrap it and someone else could eat it. You can't waste money on food like that and just throw it away."

Wow! Here we had another aspect. I walked her to the rubbish bin and said, "Now throw it in." She did but was visibly shaken. Back we went to tapping again on this new aspect. We tapped on all of the above that she had said, plus much more came up and I just tapped as she spoke.

If food is in front of you then you must eat it all. You can't have any waste. Clean your plate. Food costs money and you can't waste it. You'll be punished if you waste it. You're being greedy if you take food and don't eat it.

After several minutes and many rounds and much emotion, she calmed down. Although I didn't check her intensity initially, it was obviously 10 out of 10 and now it was down to 0. She went to the rubbish bin, looked at the ice cream, which was now melting, and said, "You'll have a nice sticky mess in there." No more emotion over waste.

She now has a tool to handle her addiction. I am in awe at the stunning simplicity of this EFT procedure.

✿ ✿ ✿

A very important element of the above session is when Dorothy asked the client to throw the Topsy away. This produced a new aspect to address with EFT, and I call that "testing the results." As I have mentioned before, when there are aspects of the issue left unaddressed, the issue will tend to come back. Whenever it seems as though the intensity is gone, find creative ways to verify that information and you will often find there is more to do.

Using EFT to address cravings directly is a great first step toward changing how you respond to food. In most cases, you can see immediate results and it is easy to see how EFT is helping you achieve your goals. However, even after EFT has been successful in eliminating one craving, or even a few cravings, any related emotional issues that have not been addressed can cause those cravings to come back in time.

For that reason, I encourage you to continue learning how to dig deeper and find the core issues behind your challenges with weight loss.

3

Food Addictions

What's the difference between a craving and an addiction? A craving is a strong desire. Cravings are usually transient. They come and go. An addiction is a long-term pattern of giving in to cravings. An addiction is an enduring behavior that persists over time. Purely physical cravings can often be easily addressed with EFT. However, addictive patterns usually aren't just physical. They're rooted in unresolved emotional trauma. Until those traumas are resolved, the addiction continues. Even if willpower succeeds in suppressing it, the addict often simply switches to a new substance.

I've worked with my share of people who no longer want their coffee, chocolate, or alcohol after one or two rounds of EFT. I've also had my share of people with seemingly endless emotional issues who truly *needed* their addictive substances or behaviors until an emotional clearing of their negative jungle occurred. It was their best solution to the problem until the causes could be eliminated. This can take time, of course.

You may notice that the cases in this chapter illustrate not only deeper emotional issues, but a higher level of experience with EFT as well. Most of these stories were submitted by experienced EFT practitioners and/or licensed therapists who have a more complete understanding of emotional issues and how to navigate through them.

I include these examples so you can see how deep the emotional issues can run, and how an experienced EFT professional might find and address them.

Improving your EFT skills will require good detective work to lead you to the specific issues that need attention, and good testing methods will let you know when there is more work to be done. You will see some great examples of both in this chapter, so feel free to try any of these approaches on your own issues.

In the first report, John Digby from the U.K. alertly uses EFT for physical symptoms that "show up" as he helps his client with a chocolate addiction.

It is always interesting to see how emotions show up as physical symptoms. People sweat when they're nervous, get a headache when they are stressed, or feel a knot in their stomach when they're scared. In this case, you will see that once the physical craving was tapped away, the emotions were still there and showed up in several physical forms.

When working on your own cravings or addictions, pay close attention to changes in your body, and be sure to address them with EFT. Because they represent aspects of the issue you are trying to resolve, they can lead you to deeper issues. Remember that even if you start by tapping on something global or general, emotional layers will be peeled away, revealing unexpected memories and very important clues for your healing process.

EFT for a Chocolate Addiction Triggers Symptoms

by John Digby

I run my practice from an office in a multi-use block of start-up companies and am opposite the kitchen, where I bump into most of the other occupants from time to time. One of the ladies that I speak with runs a local Weight Watchers group and had vouchsafed to me that she had a real addiction to *chocolate!* Now there's a surprise! Last Thursday I met her in the kitchen and this time asked her if she could spare ten minutes to see if I could help. She said okay.

We sat down and I showed her a small packet of German chocolate that I keep for demonstration purposes when running workshops. Her level of intensity was 9.5 on the 0-to-10 scale. I asked her to tap the Karate Chop point while she smelled the chocolate and described it to me. We then went onto EFT's Basic Recipe using reminder words like *smooth, yummy, warm, comforting, dribbling,* and *I really want it.* We breathed deeply and sighed. I asked for her level of intensity and she said there was none but that she felt sick.

We then did one shortcut round on feeling sick in the pit of her stomach and I asked for her level of intensity again. At this point she said she no longer felt sick but had a headache over her left eyebrow. After another short version for "sharp pain over my left eye," I asked her level of intensity again. Now she was completely clear and willing to throw the chocolate in the waste bin.

I found the diverse aspects of this five-minute session very interesting and was bowled over today when she looked in to say a heartfelt thanks. She said that since our session, she was feeling a lot more grounded and alert to the world and life in general. She really does seem a new woman, and all in five minutes. She has booked her place on my next introductory EFT workshop, and we are both looking forward to it immensely.

❅ ❅ ❅

In this next report, Dr. Carol Solomon describes a weight-related tapping session that reveals some emotional themes common among people with weight problems, like a need for approval or a need for attention. Dr. Solomon has previous experience with cases of this kind, and she is able to suggest directions for the session that beginners may not be able to replicate on their own. However, if any of these directions feel as though they fit for you, do a few similar rounds of tapping and see where they take you.

This case also illustrates more global uses of EFT, as seen in the various Setup Phrases. Global language is generally more effective if you use it with a longer term plan, and as you will see, this client tapped every day for a month and was encouraged to use EFT as a daily practice.

For faster results, this client's past issues could be broken down into specific events and the sting from these events could be "tapped away" quickly.

You will also see new aspects showing up as physical symptoms, just as we saw in the previous case. An interesting twist here is that Dr. Solomon treats them as metaphors for her client's emotional issues by suggesting that her client's family is a "pain in the neck" and that they give her a backache.

Morbidly Obese Woman Stops Feeling Hungry

by Dr. Carol Solomon

My client Jean was morbidly obese and had been unable to lose weight for many years. No matter what she tried, it would only last a short time before her eating got out of control again. Like many clients with persistent food and weight issues, Jean was holding onto old childhood hurts. She felt deprived as a child. Her mother was emotionally needy, and her sister, "the beautiful one," got most of the attention. Jean only got attention for being "responsible."

What Jean didn't get from her family, she gave to herself. Jean didn't think that she could get love and attention from her family, so she "settled" for food.

It didn't stop her from continuing to try to get her family's approval, even as an adult. Jean spent her entire life in search of the love and attention she didn't get from her family while hating herself for not being the one they gave it to. Jean's low self-esteem led to excessive pleasing behavior, in which she hid her true self while being unable to set limits. I don't know anything that will create stress more quickly than saying "yes" to everything!

Hanging onto her excess weight became a symbol for the only kind of attention Jean thought she could get. These patterns became obvious in one of my EFT sessions with her.

Even though I need to be needed...

Even though I need to show them how responsible I am...

She added:

Even though my fat gives me negative attention, and otherwise they ignore me, I love and accept myself anyway.

Even though I've spent my whole life breaking my back trying to please them.

At this point, Jean said her back started to hurt.

Even though they give me a backache...

Then the pain moved to her neck.

Even though they are a big pain in the neck, I love and accept myself completely.

Even though I can't accept that I'm not going to get the attention I want from them, I love and accept myself completely.

Even though I can't say no because they might think I'm not responsible, and that's all I have...

Even though I need to hang onto this fat to get attention, otherwise I'm invisible, I love and accept myself anyway.

Even though I'm still trying to prove myself, I approve of myself and I accept where I am in this process.

Jean's back and neck pain disappeared immediately. She tapped for a few minutes per day for about a month using a combination of these statements. I encouraged her to make EFT a daily practice. She is now steadily losing one to two pounds per week and she has stopped feeling "hungry" all the time. As a bonus, she no longer feels that she needs to say "yes" to every request and is feeling much happier.

❖ ❖ ❖

Although it seems like a nice little bonus, the change in Jean's overall behavior is one of the most powerful, yet subtle, benefits of using EFT. In many cases, we address pain, or weight loss, or some other current complaint, but by cleaning up the unresolved emotional events behind them, major shifts can happen. Eventually, the past is no longer unresolved or painful, and all of our conditioned behaviors, beliefs, and habits that we adopted in the past are no longer necessary. That's what we call emotional freedom!

The following report by Tam Llewellyn of the U.K. provides clear evidence of the link between addictions and unresolved emotional issues. His client could drink alcohol socially with no signs whatsoever of alcoholism. However, when she drank a specific brand of beer—Budweiser—her drinking of *that* beer became uncontrollable.

Much of the "comfort" we derive from "comfort foods" has similar links to the past, and putting your EFT detective skills to use in finding them may help control your appetite just as dramatically as Tam's client controlled her appetite for Budweiser.

This session begins with a very simple application of basic EFT and demonstrates some standard real-time tests to evaluate the results. Once the emotional component is revealed you will see that the Setup language clearly points to a collection of specific events in which Budweiser meant good times. To be more specific in the session, any of those individual events could be addressed with Tell the Story Technique or the Movie Technique.

After addressing the emotional component, Tam uses some positive phrasing in the Setup to reframe his client's perspective. This approach is a more advanced EFT tool, and should generally be used only after the intensity has been released, just as Tam illustrates.

Budweiser and Emotions That Cause Addictions

by Tam Llewellyn

In EFT workshops, I often ask participants to bring addictive substances if they wish to see EFT remove the addiction. These usually involve sugar, chocolate, cigarettes, and coffee. However, at a recent workshop one of the participants came up with an unusual request.

Emma was not an alcoholic, in that she could do without alcohol and did for long periods, and she could take a social drink or two and not want more. Her problem was with Budweiser beer. Once she had a bottle she could not stop drinking it. She would drink and drink and drink until no more was available. To complicate matters, Emma wanted to lose her addiction to Budweiser beer but wanted to retain her liking for an occasional beer when it suited her.

I had never been asked to remove only part of an addiction. However, being willing to try anything once and with Gary Craig's words "Try it on everything!" ringing in my ears, I started the demonstration.

When a bottle of Budweiser was placed in front her, Emma immediately reported a 0-to-10 craving of 10. We tapped together for:

Even though I have a craving for this Budweiser beer, I deeply and completely accept and love myself.

We used the Reminder Phrase "Craving for Budweiser beer" while doing a full round of tapping. That first round reduced the craving to a 5, and after the second, it fell to a 2. I cracked the bottle open and the resulting hiss immediately took the craving back to 10. More rounds reduced it again to a 4 or 5, and even sipping the beer did not increase the craving, but it did not show any signs of falling, either.

It was Emma herself who made the breakthrough. She said, *"It's not the Budweiser beer, but the happy times I have associated with it."* That changed the line of the therapy and while I continued tapping around the points, she repeated my words:

Even though I loved those times, and want them back, and Budweiser beer reminds me of them, I deeply and completely accept and love myself as I am now.

Those times were great and so was the Budweiser beer, but I do not need it now. I can still remember and enjoy those times without the Budweiser beer.

I have a film running in my head called "Those Budweiser Beer Days" and I can remember them well. They were great.

Even though I think I need Budweiser beer to help me recover those times, I deeply and completely accept and love myself.

This work brought the craving level down to 2 and even sipping it did not bring it back up again. Emma said she could do without it and that anyway it tasted "strange," but she still had a little wish for it and those happy times.

This time we tapped while saying:

Even though I may need this Budweiser beer to recall those happy times, I choose to recall and enjoy them without Budweiser beer and I will be amazed and intrigued at how easy it is for me to rerun the film of those times (now re-titled simply "Happy Days") any time I wish. It is amazing that I do not need those days to come again — I am happy as I am now and I can still have lovely memories.

The craving level was down to 0 and Emma was having uncontrolled fits of laughter.

Emma and the group were with us for a full week learning various therapies, and during that week I saw her drinking the occasional can of beer. But even when it was offered or even pressed on her, she never drank more than a sip of Budweiser, saying it was nowhere near as nice as other beers and really tasted a bit funny!

❅ ❅ ❅

Dr. Carol Solomon is up next to address an intense craving for ice cream. Once again, after peeling away a few surface layers, a very clear core issue emerges and presents an entire collection of specific events from childhood. The connection between the events and the craving is so clear that you might wonder why Jannie didn't see it sooner. However, the human emotional framework can be tricky and elusive, so it's always good to have a tool like EFT and an experienced professional like Dr. Solomon to guide you through.

Detective Work for an Ice-Cream Addiction

by Dr. Carol Solomon

I teach a three-week teleclass on "EFT for Weight Loss," and I have people bring food to the first call so we can tap for cravings in the moment. After the first round of a recent class, almost everyone's craving was down, except one woman, "Jannie."

Jannie was tapping on her craving for ice cream, although she said she didn't bring it to the call because "unless someone delivered it as I dialed in, I would have eaten it the minute it came in the house!"

We tapped for cravings:

Even though I have this craving, I deeply and completely accept myself.

Even though I really want this food right now...

Even though I have this urge to eat...

We used the Reminder Phrase "this craving" on each tapping spot.

Her craving went from a 10 to a 2. But she was still worried that if someone put a bowl of ice cream in front of her, she would eat it, or that the craving could be triggered again in a stressful situation.

So we tapped more:

Even though I don't quite want to let it go, I deeply and completely accept myself.

Even though I'm afraid I'll still want it...

Even though I have these cravings that are triggered by stress...

Even though I want things I think I shouldn't have...

We changed Reminder Phrases as we tapped the EFT points down the body, saying: *these cravings...*

triggered by stress…I can't quite release it…I'm still hanging on…It's triggered by stress…I'm afraid I might still want it….I don't quite trust it yet…

Between the first and second call, Jannie did buy a quart of ice cream. It stayed in her refrigerator for 12 hours—11 hours and 59 minutes longer than usual! When she opened it, she just ate the cherries out and threw the rest away. She hasn't purchased any since and has no desire to get any.

On the third call, we tapped for specific events. Jannie came up with five events that had an emotional charge. These specific events all occurred when she was between seven and fifteen years old, and they all had to do with her parents and with her being denied something. For tapping during the class she picked "my mother eating ice cream every evening after dinner and I was not allowed any."

Jannie's mother was a 105-pound, 5-foot 2-inch, extremely beautiful woman who took very good care of herself and her home. She loved ice cream, so every evening she'd go to the freezer, pile ice cream into her salad bowl-sized dish, curl up at the end of the sofa, and eat it slowly bite by bite.

Jannie was not allowed to have any ice cream, ever, because she was chubby and "Jannie doesn't get sweets" was a house rule.

At some point in her life, Jannie made a decision, based on her interpretation of these childhood experiences, which she described in a letter to me following the class. She wrote:

Dear Carol,

When I decide to get ice cream, I always tell myself, "I deserve it"—not as a reward for anything, I just I deserve it. I never could figure this out because I am someone who is actually more humble than this and hugely grateful for my life and all I have been given.

Carol, this is phenomenal for me. It finally makes sense, perfect sense, actually. I did deserve it when those energies were stuck in the denial from my mother. When I tapped through all those issues around ice cream (being denied, feeling I deserved it, that I could have it anytime I wanted it, accepting my mother for who she was able to be and loving her anyway), I felt a great relief. I am at 0 now with ice cream. And what I love most of all is that it finally makes sense to me! I remember that my mother always had gallons of ice cream around as well as all kinds of candy. I wondered why I didn't just go eat all that stuff anyway (I was not an obedient child). Then I remembered (funny, I had forgotten) that my parents had a lock on the freezer and a cupboard with a padlock in the kitchen to keep me out!

So I asked myself why have I never chowed down on all of those things all the time since I left home and have the freedom to do so? My eating is typically very healthy (I never keep anything in the house that is tempting to me) and although I am twenty pounds overweight, this is more due to orthopedic injuries and mid-life hormones than poor eating. In class #1, you said to me that I needed to trust myself. That resonated because, although I do really well, I strategically and stringently set up my environment to keep temptations out—always.

So my next revelation is about goodies locked up by my parents...I cannot be trusted, but I love all those goodies, so I essentially "lock up" all the goodies I'd love because I don't trust myself. So when you said I needed to trust myself, I actually felt your words in my heart right then, and now that I've figured it out, I feel such peace in knowing I can trust myself.

So Carol, this has been amazing for me and I thank you from the bottom of my heart. What I find with you is your insights and words bring normalcy to me and you make beautiful sense and connections and I feel all this so profoundly.

I thank you so much for pursuing this with me. I just read that victims will feel a sense of entitlement, and that resonates with me in thinking "I deserve this ice cream! Wow!"

In a four-month follow up, Jannie wrote to say that her results have held up, even under stressful circumstances. She tapped for a craving one more time, two weeks after the class ended. She wrote, "I must tell you that ice cream is so far out of the picture for me now. The true test has been my husband needing surgery and me needing "something" for comfort, but ice cream never even crossed my mind! I've been happily choosing berries, cherries, and grapes instead! This is an absolute miracle!!! Thank you, thank you!"

✿ ✿ ✿

Addictive cravings sometimes represent a crying out for love. You can often identify such cases when a few rounds of EFT directed at cravings have only minimal impact. That's because there's a bigger emotional need that drives them. In the next report, Gabriele Rother from Germany illustrates this concept beautifully.

Once again, global descriptions in the Setup peel away some layers so the core issue can come though. The extended Setup Phrases in the rest of the session are designed to increase the intensity of the anger by describing it in more detail. By focusing on the anger to this degree, the tapping can correct the related energy disruption more completely.

The Reminder Phrases are not distinguished from the Setup Phrases here, but you can assume that this language was used while tapping through the sequence and not just on the Karate Chop point.

Gabriele addresses several aspects along the way and then closes the session after resolving a specific event with her client's father.

A Chocolate Addiction
And the Reason Behind It

by Gabriele Rother

A woman called and asked me how she could tap for her intense craving for chocolate. She had experienced sudden attacks of cravings and was very angry at herself for eating the all of the chocolate in her possession at once.

We started tapping with the Setup Phrases:

Even though I have this ravenous appetite for chocolate, I deeply and completely accept myself.

Even though I don't like myself because I am so weak every time that I cannot resist…

Even though I am so angry afterward…

Even though I have this addiction to chocolate…

This yearning for chocolate…

"What is your real yearning?" I asked. She replied, "Craving for security."

We tapped while saying:

Even though this yearning inside myself lets me take the chocolate…Chocolate means security for me. I never felt secure. I yearn for it so badly. I yearn for it forever. I know chocolate is not the same. Chocolate only reminds me of security and feeling safe.

After that round she felt very angry, and a lot of rage came up about the fact that she wasn't protected by her parents. They both were employed and didn't have time enough for her. This made her very upset. We tapped for:

> *This rage about my parents…I am still so furious, even though this happened a long time ago. I yearned so much for security and protection. I never got it. There was nobody protecting me. I had this yearning. This yearning is still there. The chocolate calms me down for a while but it comes back. And I am so angry about myself and about my parents. I am angry!*

After this round she calmed down a bit, but it came to her that she was still angry with her aunt. She experienced abuse during a stay at her grandmother's and she told her aunt about that. But her aunt refused to listen to her and didn't take her seriously. That upset her. We tapped for:

> *Even though I feel this anger about my aunt… She didn't take me seriously. I am so angry about her. She didn't believe me. Nobody takes me seriously. That makes me so furious! I am mad with anger! But maybe my aunt was afraid of this man. I am still furious about her! Maybe she experienced something similar and had fears like me, but I am still furious…Nobody takes me seriously. But the chocolate takes me seriously. It is always there and gives me a good feeling. I wished I could have gotten that same feeling from my aunt.*

After this round the anger about the aunt was gone. Now a sort of sadness and a feeling of anger came up about her father. He refused to take her home, and she was not able to tell him what happened with this man and that made her sad and angry at same time. We tapped:

My father…He didn't take me home. I am so angry about this. He does not love me. And I wasn't able to tell him what happened. Couldn't tell it to Grandma, neither to Dad, and my aunt refused to listen. I am so sad and so angry! But Dad wanted to protect me. He wanted to do his best for me. In his view, the best thing for me was to stay with my grandma. But he didn't know what happened there. He still loves me. And I couldn't tell him. If he knew what happened, he would have taken me home. But I couldn't tell him. At least it was okay. Nothing more happened. My aunt took care of me. At the end she protected me. I can let it go now and enjoy my chocolate without longing for it. I can enjoy the chocolate without being angry. I don't need to eat it up all at once. I can enjoy it that I feel safe now even without chocolate. I am protected and I am okay like I am.

Deep breath out. All of the anger and the sadness were gone. I asked her about her longing for chocolate. It was completely gone and she felt a deep release. This session took us about a quarter of an hour.

❀ ❀ ❀

Here's a brief idea from Dr. Deborah Miller that brings about big results for stubborn food cravings. Notice how her approach involves common-sense questions.

Finding Out What
Really Caused a Food Craving

by Dr. Deborah Miller

I enjoy how EFT allows one to get to the core reason for a food craving. This interesting story shows how well we hide the reasons.

I facilitate individual sessions and group classes titled "EFT Ideal Weight." It is a delightful way to look at the myriad causes of holding onto weight.

In one particular class dealing with food cravings, each person brought an item that she had cravings for. I asked each woman to look at the food item, smell it, and sense the emotions that came to the surface because I wanted them to identify what it was about the item that they craved. Was it the look, the taste, the texture?

With EFT the craving level dropped quickly for everyone except one woman. Her craving was for a specific type of bread. When I asked her what it was about the bread that she craved she admitted that it wasn't the bread. It was dunking the bread in milk. I asked her what it was about dunking the bread in milk that she enjoyed. She told me that it made the bread soft. The type of bread she craved is dry bread commonly used for dunking in milk or hot chocolate.

Then I asked her if there was something in her life that was hard that she wanted to make soft. Her eyes got wide and she stated that her husband was sometimes hard with her and she wished he'd be softer. From that moment on her craving level for the bread dropped to nothing. Since this session she hasn't had a craving for dunking bread in milk.

❅ ❅ ❅

German EFT practitioner Horst Benesch could not get a woman beyond her cookie craving until he persisted with questions and discovered a core issue. Once the core issue was collapsed with EFT, the cookie craving disappeared. Identifying core issues is an important concept that all serious practitioners need to master. Horst uses both the Karate Chop point and the Sore Spot while doing the Setup. You'll find the Sore Spot described in Appendix A.

The Core Issue Behind a Cookie Addiction

by Horst Benesch

In a recent EFT workshop I placed cookies in the middle of the tables and asked whether anyone irresistibly had to eat one of them. A forty-two-year-old woman said she could not imagine not eating this sugar-coated cookie. I let her smell and taste a bit, and she rated her craving at a 7.

We tapped for the craving, but there was no change. It remained a 7. We switched from the Karate Chop point to the Sore Spot with more emphasis, but no change. I let her bite a small piece again and asked her to describe what she sensed. She reported a certain pleasurable sense of melting in her mouth.

Even though I like this melting feeling in my mouth…

No change, still a 7.

I then asked her to describe this melting more exactly, asking what it felt like for her. She said, *"Smooth, warm, and sweet."* And she added: *"That is because my mother never nursed me."* I wanted to hook into this argument, but she refused and said it was just a joke. Nevertheless I asked her whether or not it was true. She conceded that her mother never had nursed her.

I told her to take this "joke" seriously, because maybe that is the way her unconscious tricked her. Thus we tapped on:

Even though my mother never did nurse me and even though I therefore miss this warm, smooth, and sweet sensation within my mouth…

After a whole round of the Basic Recipe, I let her taste it again. She was astonished and reported that this cookie tasted sweeter.

Another round of tapping, again tasting. Now she reported that it tasted unpleasantly sweet and she did not want to eat this cookie anymore. As a challenge I put cookies directly in front of her during the whole evening. She did not even feel a slight desire for them.

At the end of this group session I asked her again to have a little taste. She did not like it at all because it was too sweet.

※ ※ ※

Carol Look has been a professional therapist for many years, and has an impressive record using EFT for addictions, weight loss, and the like. Over the years, she has identified several emotional "themes" that often contribute to addiction and weight loss, and in this case, we learn about grief.

In her article below, Carol tells us about how she addressed cravings at a workshop with a group of volunteers. Coincidentally, or maybe not, several of these volunteers had unresolved grief in their past. Once these stories are revealed by her volunteers, you can see how one traumatic event, left unresolved, can translate in to a lifetime of eating habits.

When applying EFT to several people at once, you often have to keep it global or general, and you may see that in Carol's Setup Phrases. This article can serve as a great illustration of how emotional issues connect to cravings, but as a follow-up on any of these issues, I would focus on the actual event of the loss with each volunteer.

Using the Client's Cravings

by Carol Look

Brenda attended my "EFT for Anxiety Relief" class at the National Guild of Hypnotists convention. As part of the agenda, I asked for volunteers for an in-class demonstration for food cravings and underlying feelings. Brenda was one of four volunteers.

She chose a bag of M&Ms from my pile of props and rated her craving for them as an 8 on the 0-to-10 point scale. Our first round of tapping was:

Even though I have these cravings, and I really love the way my favorite food tastes, I deeply and completely accept myself.

Each person's 0-to-10 craving rating decreased. One woman said her craving had gone down significantly and she was now thinking of the good times she had with her father. Brenda echoed this thought and reported feeling profound grief. She had lost her father when she was eight years old and her mother couldn't handle Brenda's grief and crying, so she gave Brenda food to shut her up.

All four volunteers associated their eating of junk foods with losses they had experienced.

Even though I feel deep grief, and I want to eat to cover it up, I deeply and completely accept myself.

Even though I feel these deep losses, and I want to stuff myself with food, I deeply and completely accept myself anyway.

Even though I feel abandoned because they left me, I deeply and completely accept my feelings.

The volunteers continued to unravel layers of sadness around the losses they had experienced. Brenda said that her craving for the M&Ms was going down dramatically, but her feelings of sadness were surfacing strongly. She told the class she had lost two children, a fiancé, and her favorite pet. She also reported having strong physical feelings of grief in her chest, which she described as "a bowling ball in my chest."

Even though I use the sweets to feel better, because I love how they make me feel, I choose to feel safe and comfortable without them.

Even though I can't get satisfied, I love myself anyway.

Even though sweets are the only things that make me feel better, I deeply and completely accept myself.

Brenda told the class that the "bowling ball feeling" in her chest, a heartache, was decreasing in intensity and moving down towards her solar plexus.

Even though I have suffered so many losses, I choose to feel accepting of myself and of them.

Even though I just want to be acknowledged for all my losses and how hard it's been, I deeply and completely love and accept my feelings.

Brenda said this one really "hit" her hard. She realized that all she had wanted was to be acknowledged for all the pain that she had been through. She told the class that everyone sees her as such a strong person and that they assume things come easily to her.

We tapped several more rounds on grief and being acknowledged.

We also tapped for Brenda's belief that whenever she gets close to someone, "they drop dead." Brenda said this last round released the tremendous pain she had been carrying around for so long. She heard herself say, *"You're right. I've suffered enough,"* and she felt free to let go of her deep grief at this point.

I talked to Brenda four weeks later to see how she was. She had been doing her own tapping during the first week but then stopped. She had not eaten any sweets since the class, including while she was on a week-long vacation in Florida. Ice cream used to be her favorite comfort food, and she hadn't had any in four weeks. On her birthday the week before she took one bite of birthday cake and didn't like it because it tasted too sweet! While in the class demonstration, Brenda used the bag of M&Ms as a symbol for all sweets in her life and was pleased that it had obviously worked for cake and ice cream as well.

Brenda said she had not gotten on the scale yet, but that several people told her she looked as if she had lost some weight.

She is ready now to deal fully with her weight issue and reported that the tapping came at exactly the right time in her life.

❊ ❊ ❊

There is a suggestion here that the results achieved in the workshop described above were more of a "good start" than a "miracle cure" and that Brenda should continue tapping. This is often the case when using global Setup Phrases instead of uncovering the specific events.

Here is another example of how an experience of grief or loss can eventually contribute to unhealthy eating habits. This next article by Melissa Derasmo is a must-read because it superbly illustrates how finding a core issue can collapse even the most stubborn challenges.

Her process provides a very good example of how everyday people without therapy experience can find their own underlying isues. Melissa immediately "got" that past events in her life were affecting her life in the present, so she committed herself completely without expecting any specific result right away. Once she was relieved of some baggage, she was able to tune into to the deeper issue comning forward.

Also notice the extent to which she tested her own results. Testing methods can dig up even more aspects and help you be much more thorough with EFT. As she discovers, it may be that one needs to tap on *what didn't happen* as well as what did.

EFT and My Sugar Addiction

by Melissa Derasmo

I was a confirmed sugar addict. Starting in my early twenties, I ate sugar at every opportunity. I would do anything I had to in order to get my "fix," including things I would rather not admit to, like stealing money if I didn't have any for chocolate or other sugar-rich things.

In a continuing effort to find the perfect diet, I somehow managed to discover EFT in August of 2007. I dove in and never looked back. I tapped for every single issue I could find, and I had a lot. I had inconsolable grief over my alcoholic mother dying when I was six, anger over being physically abused by a stepmother and sexually abused by *her* father, and then inconsolable grief over my father passing away when I was ten years old. These were big issues, but I was able to eliminate all their pain with EFT. I spent the next year working on my Personal Peace Procedure and tapping on everything I could come up with. But I still ate sugar uncontrollably.

Then on February 1, 2009, something happened that started me down the road to the answer. I was in Macy's shopping (which was my second favorite thing to do at that time) and suddenly out of nowhere a baby started screaming and crying. Well, my reaction to that was to get out of the room as fast as possible. My husband, who was with me at the time, turned to me and said, *"What is wrong with you?"* And it hit me. I thought *everyone* runs out of the room when there's a crying baby. I can't tolerate hearing babies cry. But no, apparently lots of people don't have this issue at all! And slowly the thought "bubbled up" for me—I can't tolerate the crying baby because *I* am the crying baby—the baby that wasn't taken care of—both while my mother was alive and after she died. So I went home and started to tap. This was a long session of working on every single thing I could come up with, and whether it was true or not did not matter. These thoughts were what I *believed* to be true.

Even though I'm so sad that my mother was too drunk to wake up and feed me...

too drunk to wake up and change my diapers...

too drunk to take care of me...

But more importantly, I realized that after she died she wasn't there to do all the things a daughter needs in life—and as I focused on what we had missed together, the tears came flooding out:

Even though I'm so sad my mother wasn't there to walk me to school,

> *tuck me in at night,*
>
> *read me a story,*
>
> *help me with my homework,*
>
> *put my picture on the fridge,*
>
> *congratulate me on my wonderful report card,*
>
> *push me on the swing in the park,*
>
> *listen to my heart aches,*
>
> *play with me,*
>
> *take me for my first bra,*
>
> *make cookies with me,*
>
> *tell me what a Tampax is,*
>
> *help me plan my wedding,*
>
> *tell me why I shouldn't marry that idiot,*
>
> *hold her first granddaughter,*
>
> *tell me what a great daughter I am,*
>
> *…and lots, lots more.*

What happened when it was all done was quite stunning. The first thing I noticed was total silence— the voice that would constantly scream out for sugar was completely silent. So I started to test. At work

I walked by my co-worker's office and the ton of chocolate on her desk — *nothing*. I went by the vending machines — *nothing*. I went to the supermarket and walked down candy aisle — *nothing*. I picked up some chocolate, smelled it, had zero desire for it, put it down, and walked away. If you are a sugar addict, you will understand that that was nothing less than a miracle. The next morning I thought perhaps I had been abducted by aliens and exchanged for an addiction-free person — someone who is "normal." I was quite unsettled about it but willing to accept that whatever happened, it was good. And while it hasn't been a terribly long time, I remain completely addiction-free weeks later. The endless, relentless "pull" that would force me to eat is completely gone. Today I eat "normally" — I make low-calorie balanced meals and I'm perfectly okay with them. I'm happy with one serving. I can watch others eat cake, cookies, and candy without any issue at all. It doesn't bother me. I simply don't want what they have.

Looking back, I can see the clue my subconscious was trying to give me with the crying baby who was always there. I didn't understand what it meant so I just ignored it. And as I now lose weight effortlessly, I hope that others will find this information useful. It may be that one needs to tap on *what didn't happen* as well as what did.

Since first collapsing the "baby crying" issue, I have now been three months without any sugar cravings and I have lost 38 pounds.

* * *

Melissa discovered both physical and sexual abuse in her past, which are very traumatic experiences that often lead to overeating. However, don't assume that only abuse survivors can relate to her process. Believe it or not, many people have been just as traumatized by a playground humiliation or by being dumped by a first love. If it was really painful for you, it can still be affecting you, so tap on whatever memories show up.

4

Are You Getting the
Results You Want?

You've now had several experiences with EFT. You've tried it on some of your cravings and probably had immediatge success. You've also probably identified some of the specific events that contributed to your eating behavior. You might have unearthed some of your limiting beliefs. Here are some guidelines for where to go next.

Results and Refinements

There are five possible outcomes after doing a full round of EFT.

1. The craving or discomfort level improves or goes away completely.

2. The location of a physical symptom, such as a headache or other pain, moves to another part of the body, even if it only moves an inch or two.

3. The quality of the craving or discomfort changes.

4. The craving or discomfort level increases.

5.   Nothing happens.

I'll cover what to do about each of these possibilities in detail, but please note that:

All of the changes in items 1 through 4 are evidence that EFT is working for you.

1. What should you do if the craving or discomfort level improves or goes away completely? If the craving or discomfort goes away completely, you are done. You're one of our well-known "one-minute wonders," and while you may find it surprising, this is a frequent occurrence. Enjoy the results and get on with your life.

If the craving or discomfort improves but doesn't go to 0, do more EFT rounds until it reaches 0 or plateaus at some improved level. If it plateaus and three or four more EFT rounds don't result in relief, you can assume that "nothing more will happen" and go to item 5 below.

If the craving or discomfort disappears but resurfaces at another time, this is evidence that more EFT is necessary. It would be a mistake to conclude that EFT "didn't work" because it obviously did. Our bodies give us many valuable messages (if we are listening) and sometimes a single symptom can have several causes. You can try more rounds of standard EFT and, eventually, the discomfort or craving may subside permanently. If not, just assume that "nothing more will happen" and go to item 5 below.

2. What should you do if the location of a physical symptom moves to another part of the body, even if it only moves an inch or two? Sometimes while tapping for a specific food craving, a person will suddenly feel nauseated or develop a headache or feel pain or discomfort somewhere in the body. (See an example on pages 95–96). Any new symptom or movement of a symptom is cause for optimism because it suggests that the original problem has been alleviated in favor of a new discomfort that now gets your attention. It could also mean that the original discomfort had an emotional cause that was "alleviated in the background" and the new discomfort or craving is evidence of a new emotional cause. In either case, start over with EFT at the new location just as though it is a brand new condition—because it is.

If the symptom moves again, then keep "chasing" it until the discomfort level falls to 0. If you get stuck on a symptom that doesn't move or if you don't get relief after three or four diligent rounds of EFT, then assume that "nothing more will happen" and proceed to item 5 below.

3. What should you do if the quality of the symptom changes from, let's say, a sharp pain to a dull ache, or from a throb to a tingle…and so on? This is similar to item 2 above except the symptom changes nature or quality instead of location. Any such quality change is cause for optimism because it suggests that the original condition has been altered.

In this case, start over with EFT as though this altered version is a new condition. Keep doing EFT rounds on any future altered symptoms until the discomfort level falls to 0. If you get stuck on an altered symptom that doesn't move or if you don't get relief on it after three or four diligent rounds of EFT, then assume that "nothing more will happen" and proceed to item 5 below.

4. What should you do if the discomfort level or craving increases? Although it doesn't happen often, I have certainly seen cases where such levels increased after one or two rounds of EFT. Many healing responses triggered by other therapies show signs of getting worse (they call it a "healing crisis") before getting better.

Three or four more rounds of EFT will usually "turn the corner" and launch noticeable relief. If not, or if the relief plateaus at a level above 0, then assume that "nothing more will happen" and proceed to item 5.

5. What should you do if nothing happens? The high likelihood here is that unresolved emotional issues are major contributors to the craving or discomfort you feel.

So now we need to search for emotional factors and apply EFT to them. Since we have so many differing emotional histories, this bit of detective work has to be customized to you. I usually do this by asking questions. Here's one:

> *If there was a specific emotional event contributing to this craving or this feeling of discomfort, what could it be?*

The beautiful thing about this question is that it often points to a vital emotional cause even if it doesn't seem that way at first. Your system has a way of knowing what is going on even if you see no realistic link. For example, your craving for vanilla pudding may seem to have no connection to the memory of your third grade teacher ridiculing you in front of the class. That's okay, just use EFT on that memory with a Setup Phrase like:

Even though Mrs. Johnson humiliated me in third grade…

Do this for as many rounds as it takes to bring your current emotional intensity on this event down to 0. When finished, you are likely to notice complete relief from the craving. If not, ask the question again and use EFT on the resulting emotional issue. Repeated efforts at this are likely to have two benefits: the emotional events will lose their sting (probably permanently) and your craving or discomfort should fade considerably.

Another good question is:

If you could live your life over again, what person or event would you just as soon skip?

This question is more general than the previous one but its answer usually leads to important specific events that need collapsing. For example, if your answer to the above is "My brother Jake," then you can break down your experience with Jake into all the specific events you have had with him that left you feeling angry, frustrated, afraid, etc.

With these two questions, you can uncover and resolve important issues that limit your life and cause you pain and/or other symptoms. That's very useful.

One point, though. You *must* come up with an answer to these questions or they will be useless. A response like

"I don't know" is unacceptable. If you really don't know, use the first guess that comes to mind. If you don't even have a guess, then *make one up!*

Often a made-up issue is as good as or better than a real one. That's because it still came from within your mind and therefore drew from material that's part of your actual experience. It still has your experiences and emotions embedded within it and it can even blend several forgotten issues together in a useful way.

When EFT Doesn't Work

When progress with EFT seems stopped—or it seems as though it doesn't work—EFT itself is usually not the problem. Rather, the reason for the lack of progress can most often be traced to the user's inexperience.

Why do I say this? Because those who master EFT don't miss very often.

They not only get their share of "one minute wonders" but impressive progress is also made for just about any problem with an emotional cause, including many physical ailments.

In those cases where the masters are stumped, however, they don't point the finger at EFT for "not working." Rather, the masters ask themselves questions like:

> *"What's in the way here?"*
>
> *"What have I not seen yet?"*
>
> *"What core issue have I been unable to find?"*

After asking myself those questions, session after session, for many years now, here is a list of the most common reasons why EFT hasn't produced the expected results.

- The problem is being approached too globally.
- The Setup was not performed completely enough.
- You have switched aspects (and may be unaware of the improvement on the previous aspect).
- You may need help from a friend or professional with a different perspective.
- You may need the Full Basic Recipe including the 9 Gamut Procedure and EFT's finger points (see Appendix A).
- You may need more instruction, so consider EFT trainings, books and DVDs.

By far, the most common reason, especially with beginners, is that the problem is being approached too globally. Next, I have included one of my tutorials from the EFT website with further insight on being as specific as possible and finding those individual events.

The Importance of Being Specific

During EFT workshops, we emphasize the importance of finding specific events to tap on. We drive home the point that a focus on specific events is critical to success in EFT. In order to release old patterns of emotion and behavior, it's vital to identify and correct the specific events that gave rise to those problems. When you hear people say, "I tried EFT and it didn't work," the chances are good that they were tapping on generalities, instead of specifics.

An example of a generality is "self-esteem" or "depression" or "performance problems." These aren't specific events. Below these generalities you'll find a collection of specific events. The person with low self-esteem might have been coloring a picture at the age of 4, when her mother walked in and criticized her for drawing outside the lines. She might have had another experience of a school teacher scolding her for playing with her hair during class during second grade, and a third experience of her first boyfriend deciding to ask another girl to the school dance.

Together, those specific events contribute to the global pattern of low self-esteem. The way EFT works is that when the emotional trauma of those individual events is resolved, the whole pattern of low self-esteem can shift. If you tap on the big pattern, and forget the specific events, you're likely to have limited success.

When you think about how the big pattern like low self-esteem is established, this makes sense. It's built up out of many single events. Collectively, they form the whole pattern. The big pattern doesn't spring to life fully formed; it's built up gradually out of many similar experiences. The memories engraved in your brain are of individual events; one disappointing or traumatic memory at a time is encoded in your memory banks. When enough similar memories have accumulated, their commonalities combine to create a common theme like "poor self-esteem." Yet the theme originated as a series of specific events, and that's where EFT can be effectively applied.

Below a generality like, "My mother didn't nurture me," you're bound to find a whole slew of individual events. One of these might be mother saying, when she was planning your sixth birthday, "You're too fat to eat cake. No more than one piece." Another might be her saying, when you were eleven, and just entering puberty, "You'll never attract a man unless you skinny up." Cumulatively, these give you the message that your mother didn't nurture you. You might today fail to nurture yourself, internalizing your mother's behavior. Yet this general problem has its roots in those very specific events.

The good news is that you don't have to tap on every single event that contributed to the global theme. Usually, once a few of the most disturbing memories have lost their emotional impact, the whole pattern disappears. Memories that are similar lose their impact once the most vivid memories have been neutralized with EFT.

Tapping on global issues is the single most common mistake newcomers make with EFT. Using lists of tapping phrases from a web site or a book, or tapping on generalities, is far less effective than tuning into the events that contributed to your global problem, and tapping on them. If you hear someone say, "EFT doesn't work," the chances are good they've been tapping globally rather than identifying specific events.

Don't make this elementary mistake. List the events, one after the other, that stand out most vividly in your mind when you think about the global problem. Tap on each of them, and you'll usually find the global problem diminishing of its own accord. This is called the "generalization effect," and it's one of the key concepts in EFT. As we tap on a painful memory and our SUD score goes down, the benefit generalizes to other similar events. Our SUD for these might reduce even though we haven't tapped on them.

Weight Loss and Tail-enders

Another way to uncover important issues, limiting beliefs, and specific events related to your weight is to use an affirmation process that will trigger "tail-enders." Tail-enders are the "yes, but" statements that contradict and sabotage your new goals.

For example, if you ask your system to confirm something that isn't currently true, such as, "I now look like a swimsuit model," your mind will instantly begin screaming its objections. Here's how to take advantage of these objections and make them work for you.

When I began my weight loss journey, I took a hard look at my routine. I'd go into the bathroom each morning, take a look at the Humpback whale around my belly, and say, "My natural weight is 222 pounds" However, I had all kinds of other voices that made contradictory statements. Those contrary voices are why affirmations don't work.

I think affirmations can be very powerful and useful, but most of us have, like me, had mixed success with them. That's because of all the tail-enders that arise when we state our affirmations. Just stating an affirmation usually brings up a host of negative voices ready to speak up and ensure we don't meet our goals.

For example, if your goal weight is 125 pounds, you might use the following statement:

My normal weight is 125 pounds and that's what I weigh.

Try this now by filling the blank with your ideal weight and saying it out loud with as much conviction as you can muster:

My normal weight is _____ pounds and that's what I weigh.

Now listen to what happens on the inside. When you declare a reality that is not currently true, your conflicting issues will often present some opposition, also known as negative self-talk or tail-enders. You might hear something like:

No way…look at the scale.
It isn't safe to be that thin.
I'm afraid of being hungry.
My friends or family won't like me.
I won't be able to complain anymore.
I can't afford new clothes.
I don't trust skinny people.
I'll never lose weight.
I'll always be fat.
I can never be skinny.

Look at this cellulite!

Losing weight is just too difficult.

Unaddressed, tail-enders have the power to sabotage any goal you try to achieve. On the bright side, tail-enders also point directly to issues you can disarm with EFT, thus removing their power from your weight loss process.

For example, if the tail-ender you heard was "My friends won't like me," you can bet there have been events in your life that helped you come to that conclusion. Take some time to review your experiences and tap on any events that might be related. Maybe your mother made fun of the skinny kid who lived next door or you heard your friends judge thin people on TV. Anything like this could contribute to your resistance to losing weight, but using EFT for those events can release their intensity and provide the freedom you need to reach your goal.

Once you identify a specific event that may be contributing to your issue with weight, simply tap the points while telling the story of that event until its emotional intensity disappears. To be more effective, identify which emotions you experienced during the event and address them individually:

Even though I felt humiliated when my mother said that, I deeply and completely accept myself.

Use *"this humiliation"* as your Reminder Phrase.

Once the emotional intensity for *humiliation* is released, substitute anger, hopelessness, or any other feeling you experienced and address it next.

There are several common "themes" for people who can't lose weight. For some, weight is a shield that protects them from having to do certain things, like socializing or being intimate. Others have a painful association with exercise or feeling hungry. Most often, for myself included, food can be a form of self-medication, something we indulge in the way other people indulge in cigarettes, alcohol, or other addictions. We do it because it makes us feel better—at least temporarily—by relieving or suppressing at least some of our stress, anxiety, fear, anger, or other damaging emotions. If any of these themes resonate with you, use them to identify the individual events that are still affecting you and address them with EFT.

Another way to find core issues is to ask yourself the simple question:

> *If there were an emotional reason why I can't lose weight, what would it be?*

You can also complete the following sentences:

> *If I reach my goal weight of 130 pounds, the consequences would be _____.*

> *In order to lose that much weight I would have to _____.*

> *Losing weight would be nice, but what I really want is _____.*

> *Losing weight reminds me of _____.*

These queries can bring up a whole daisy chain of events, beliefs, attitudes, and other tail-enders that are restricting your life and showing up on your body as excess pounds. Whether you use challenging questions, affirmations, or some other process to find these issues, break them down into specific events and tap them away with EFT. You'll notice a greater sense of overall relief with each event you address and soon your excess need for food will start to fade.

More Helpful Hints

If your issue is stubborn and just won't budge, or if you are ready for even better results, here are some more approaches you can try.

- **Tap with a friend:** Whether it's the feeling of support, an objective outside perspective, or the increased motivation, tapping with a friend can often make a big difference in your results. Find a friend who also wants to lose weight and then schedule an hour together once or twice a week. Work together to find the underlying events, then take turns using the Tell the Story Technique to address them.

- **Break out the oldies and the photo albums:** What are your favorite songs from the "good old days"? Do you remember any that still make you cry? What about the yearbooks and old family photos? Chances are, your old collections of music and photographs will remind you of important emotional events that you might overlook otherwise.

- **Adding emphasis:** When your normal tapping rounds haven't shown any progress, try raising your voice to add some emphasis. Shout the Setup Phrase, especially the "I deeply and completely accept myself" part. Say it with as much emotion as possible and see if that makes a difference.

- **What words are you using?** If you feel intimidated because you're unsure of what words to use, then it's likely that you are not being specific enough. Ask yourself a few more questions and do a little more detective work. Once you find something specific, like an event from the past, then use the Tell the Story Technique and just describe it as though you were telling it to a friend. Otherwise, go back to the default "Even though I have this _____, I deeply and completely accept myself."

- **Testing, testing, testing:** Whether you're working on a craving or a more general belief about food, putting yourself in the actual situation is a very powerful way to dig up contributing factors. What are the times of day, emotional events, or particular foods that make you feel the most like eating? In those moments, try *not eating* and take a few moments to see what emotions or memories are there waiting for you. Going to your parents' house for dinner might also bring up childhood food memories that need attention.

- **Daily tapping:** If all of this detective work and bothersome memories are more than you want to deal with right now, just try tapping every day. You can tap on whatever emotional events happen during the day, or just do a few rounds on "Even though I have this weight loss issue…" It is a global, longer-term approach, but if you tap your meridian points several times a day for a month, you may be surprised by the results.

- **Personal Peace Procedure:** I always recommend the Personal Peace Procedure as a fantastic way to start making significant shifts in your life. Rather than doing all the detective work, you can sit down once and make a list of past events that were less than pleasant. Then simply resolve one or more each day with EFT. The complete instructions were provided in Chapter 1.

- **Easy EFT:** This is a tap-along procedure that you can use with EFT videos. Just identify a problem that you want to work on, choose one of the free Tap-Along Videos on EFT Universe, and tap along with the session. You can do this once a day or as often as you like. The sessions are entertaining and you get to "borrow benefits" for yourself. Please review the complete instructions in Appendix B before getting started.

- **Hire a practitioner:** The EFT Universe website provides a list of certified EFT professionals who resolve these issues for a living. Many of them list weight loss as a specialty, but you will get good results from anyone who can uncover your core issues. Keep in mind that EFT is just as effective over the phone or Skype, so I would suggest working with one who seems best suited for you, rather than the one located closest to you.

The following case from Michelle Hardwick shows how easily tapping can be worked into your daily routine.

Sugar Cravings Subside with Persistent EFT

by Michelle Hardwick

I encourage all my clients to use EFT on a regular basis. This allows them to feel empowered and to be in charge of their own growth, change, and healing and to have the tools to continue to make changes throughout the rest of their lives. I encourage everyone to tap. I tell them that I tap in the car, when on the toilet, in the shower, waiting for planes/trains/buses etc., in fact *anywhere!* I give plenty of examples so that clients can see how EFT can be a part of their everyday lives, not just once a week or fortnight when they see an EFT practitioner!

Recently, I encouraged one of my clients, who was suffering from extreme sugar cravings that were completely out of control, to tap on a regular basis, whenever she thought of sugar, whenever she thought of overeating, whenever the urge or craving hit, during it, after it if she forgot to tap, and whenever she felt fearful or worried about a craving happening again in the future. I asked her to think about as many other aspects about the craving that she could think of and tap on them. I explained that the more specific she could be in that moment about the craving, the better.

She returned for a follow-up session this week, saying, "Wow! It really works! I tapped during the ad breaks while watching TV. I just put the TV on mute and did a good couple of rounds of tapping and when my program came back on, I turned the sound back on and continued watching. There's not a night I didn't do that tapping."

And what happened to her sugar craving? She went 13 days without feeling it at all! That same craving had been out of control for the past five weeks. We still have a little way to go, but we made major progress after just one session! She was thrilled with the change.

So for those of you who say there's not enough time in your day to tap, I suggest that you first tap on the belief of having "no time to tap," and how about doing it during your ad breaks? Happy tapping!!

❊ ❊ ❊

5

Exploring Underlying Issues

Every once in a while, someone tries the basic EFT formula and gets immediate, lasting results. The problem disappears in a single session and never comes back. One-minute wonders can and do happen, even with overwhelming cravings and an inability to lose weight. But in many cases, at some point after basic EFT reduces or eliminates a symptom or problem, it comes back. If this happens to you, don't assume that EFT didn't work. EFT worked fine for the problem you treated, but now a new aspect has presented itself, which just means there's more to do.

In this next example, Tam Llewellyn of the U.K. helps a woman lose weight when he discovers an aspect that she wasn't aware of.

Finding the Root of the Problem

by Tam Llewellyn

When we use EFT it is essential that we tap on the correct problem. This may seem obvious, but it is very easy to miss the major aspect of the problem — the one which is really driving the discomfort.

Finding the "correct" Setup Phrase is essential. I feel that when EFT fails to solve the issue, by far the most likely reason is that we have chosen the wrong aspect of the problem, or even the wrong problem altogether. Often the problem seems obvious, but in these cases we should be especially on our guard. If it is so obvious, why was it not identified and treated long ago?

In a case that illustrates this point, a middle-aged woman had a number of physical and emotional problems that all appeared to relate to her being grossly overweight. The cause of her excess weight was obvious — she ate too much and exercised too little.

We worked on various aspects of her over-eating and found that they were all related to incidents in her past. These were soon dealt with using EFT and her weight dropped a little. However, she eventually admitted to being "hooked" on Crunchie Bars (a chocolate bar available in U.K.). Her craving for them was removed using EFT to the extent that the smell and very idea of them revolted her. The job appeared to be done and I left a month's gap until her next appointment, expecting her to lose a considerable amount of weight by then and to be ready to work with me on other problems.

But a month later she returned, still overweight and still eating Crunchie Bars. She hated the smell and taste of the Crunchie Bars but was still eating four or five a day! We spent a long session exploring this aspect and I eventually discovered that many years ago the client had been in a "Weight Watchers' Club" using a strict diet plan. Crunchie Bars were included in the diet as a reward if one complied with the diet. They had been associated in the client's mind as a reward and she still felt happy and rewarded eating them—even though they tasted awful!

We could have tapped forever on her excessive weight and the problems it was causing, but we would likely have gotten little result. As soon as the link between Crunchie Bars and the feeling of reward was tapped away, her weight and related problems disappeared.

❖ ❖ ❖

While this next article by Janet Smith doesn't go into specific EFT tapping details, it does an excellent job of getting behind the type of issues that cause people to carry extra weight. It also describes how EFT success stories can inspire students and practitioners alike in their use of EFT for problem solving.

Persistent EFT for Chubby Issues

by Janet Smith

I have always had a serious propensity for all foods sweet and creamy—and a reputation for having an unquenchable appetite for such things. Even when I was able to temporarily eliminate my sugar addiction through EFT last year, I always seemed to sabotage myself by indulging in ice cream or chocolate. So, when I read an article in the EFT newsletter about the core issue behind a woman's cookie craving (the fact that her mother had never nursed her), a big light bulb went off! My mother had tried to nurse me but wasn't able to. Unfortunately, she didn't realize this until I lost a lot of weight and became rather emaciated. I was horribly unhappy and colicky, and it wasn't until I was put on formula that I became a happier and (very) chubby baby.

As long as I can remember, I have struggled with my weight and my love of sweets. I decided to try EFT on my similar issue, linking it to the idea that I associate sweet and creamy foods with the comfort and security I never got as a baby because I was starving and denied the food I so desperately needed. However, that didn't seem to work. In fact, over the course of the two days after I applied EFT, I actually craved sweet flavors and creaminess even more than I had in the recent past! I couldn't figure out what was going on, but I went back to *The EFT Manual* and started to read about Psychological Reversal. It made sense as the reason for my stalled progress, but what could I do about it?

I suddenly realised that the sweet and creamy cravings were also connected to my ongoing body weight issue — I work out intensively at the gym five or six days a week and have significantly increased my muscle mass, but my metabolism has remained stubbornly sluggish, and I have lost very little fat regardless of my workouts. I became conscious that many people in my life — family, teachers, friends — had always called me smart, not athletic.

The message I received was that I could never be lean, strong, and beautiful. I started to tap on that, and feelings rose to the surface, one after the other. First, I started laughing about the silly people telling me these things. Then I started to feel really angry! What right did they have to pigeonhole me into not being the "athletic type"? To always remember me as being chubby (and comment on it when they saw me after a few years away), even when they'd seen me thin at other times in my life? Vivid memories about my mother telling me how beautiful I could have looked in my prom dress — "if you could just lose five more pounds, it would be perfect." I started shouting as I tapped, and my eyes started to tear, thinking about all the hurt that those statements had done to me over the years. And then suddenly that started to fade, and I started to embrace the idea that I could be lean, strong, and beautiful.

I could erase those harmful words and forgive all the people who had contributed them. I started to smile and feel strong and confident in myself, and the best part was the overall sense of relief I was starting to feel. While I had already embraced that I am very strong, I could finally imagine my body being lean, and I could imagine feeling beautiful because of it, which is an image I had never been able to tangibly visualize before.

By the time I finished, I was feeling lighter, I was smiling, and I was barely able to picture a piece of chocolate in my mind!

❋ ❋ ❋

The Comfort Zone

The *comfort zone* is a critical concept within all performance pursuits. This is the mental range in which you subconsciously believe you belong. Your comfort zone is what keeps a behavior its current level and, without properly addressing it, any improvements you might achieve may not last.

Like a thermostat that keeps a room within a comfortable temperature range, our experience fluctuates within certain comfort zones. Ironically, most comfort zones aren't really comfortable, especially when we want to make changes. It's more accurate to call them *familiar* zones.

To properly enhance one's performance, condition, or situation, two factors should be addressed.

1. You must move the boundaries of your comfort zone, and

2. You must address the specific impediments to performance that need improvement.

Here are some examples of Setup Phrases that can help people involved in many different activities move beyond their present comfort zones. Please note that they all include a statement about the new or desired level of performance, whether it's an improved golf score, better grades, or the person's income. This is important in order to move mentally into a new vision of themselves.

> *Even though I'm not comfortable at the thought of golfing in the high 70s and may think I don't belong there, I deeply and completely accept myself.*

> *Even though I think I am capable of being an A student in math but have never been above a B yet...*

> *Even though the violin doesn't dance in my hands like it does in my dreams...*

> *Even though I have yet to earn $200,000 per year...*

> *Even though, as a speaker, I feel uptight and have yet to have fun with my audience...*

> *Even though I just don't feel attractive and don't have the same outgoing charisma as [pick a role model]...*

> *Even though I go "gulp" instead of flowing freely when I try to sing that high note in [name a song]...*

> *Even though writer's block seems to be always with me instead of ideas flowing out of me like a fountain...*

These go on endlessly and, of course, you must customize your approach to fit the situation. The idea is to move to a new mental image of yourself in which you see yourself as "belonging" at this new level.

Truly skilled EFT artists do a thorough job with their clients' comfort zones. They dig for the *specific events* underlying their clients' less-than-optimum performance levels and use EFT to obliterate these barriers.

When it comes to weight loss, your comfort zone is the weight range you usually maintain. It is easy for most people to lose a little weight, but when the weight loss goal is substantial, it's often outside the person's comfort zone. When that happens, self-sabotage enters the picture and the subconscious mind conspires with energy blocks, tail-enders, and negative self-talk to prevent the desired weight loss.

One way to use EFT to expand your weight-loss comfort zone is to choose a goal weight that is (as far as your mind is concerned) within the realm of possibility. Just as a golfer whose usual score is over 100 will find it hard to imagine shooting in the low 60s, someone who is 100 pounds overweight will find it hard to imagine easily reaching his or her goal weight.

But if the golfer sets a more modest goal, like shooting in the low 90s or high 80s, and if the overweight person decides to lose 20 or 30 pounds rather than 100 pounds, the subconscious mind is more likely to cooperate and less likely to generate self-sabotage. Many weight-loss success stories began with modest goals that, once achieved, led to revised and more ambitious goals. That's why I personally started with 40 pounds, knowing that I would probably need to lose more later.

EFT Setups that can help expand your weight-loss comfort zone include:

*Even though I can't imagine ever being a size 12
again, I deeply and completely accept myself.*

*Even though it's been a long time since I weighed 150
pounds, I would like to love and forgive my body and my
past food choices.*

*Even though I have yet to lose five pounds, let alone
25 or 50, I deeply and completely accept myself anyway.*

*Even though it will be easier for me to climb stairs
and get the exercise I need if I lose weight, I can move
forward in a new direction starting now.*

*Even though I haven't been in a swimsuit for years,
and the thought of wearing one in public is a real stretch,
I would love to start swimming again.*

*Even though I'm not used to thinking of weight-loss
as effortless or enjoyable, I know that with EFT, just
about anything is possible.*

Whenever you incorporate a goal into your EFT
Setup Phrases, be on the alert for tail-enders, the "yes,
but" statements that interfere with your progress. As soon
as they come to mind, follow them back to specific events
and the core issues they created. Becoming an EFT detective will help you quickly and efficiently clear away the
mental and energy blocks that can otherwise undermine
your best-laid plans.

Detective Skills

Core issues behind weight gain and cravings are often
clever about hiding, so being a good detective is an EFT

asset. Finding them can be as simple as asking yourself a few good questions:

What does this craving remind me of?

When was the first time I felt this way? And what was happening in my life at that time?

If there is a deeper emotion underlying this situation, what might it be?

Who or what is behind my weight gain?

If I could live my life over again, what person or event would I prefer to skip?

If there were a consequence for losing weight, what would it be?

If there were a benefit to keeping the weight, what would it be?

How do I feel just before I get the munchies? Exhausted, stressed, frustrated, sad, empty, angry, insecure, alone, disappointed...? And what does that feeling remind me of?

Once you have an answer to any of these questions, continue asking *"Why?"* or *"What's behind that?"* until you find unresolved specific events.

If you can't think of anything, you can try a few rounds of EFT on something global to remove a few emotional layers and see if anything new pops up.

Even though I have this weight issue and I don't know what is causing it, I deeply and completely accept myself.

For Reminder Phrases try *"This weight issue"* or *"Whatever is causing my weight issue."*

> *Even though food makes me feel better and I don't understand why, I deeply and completely accept myself.*

For Reminder Phrases try *"Food makes me feel better"* and/or *"I wonder why."*

> *Even though I eat when I'm not hungry, and I know there is an emotional cause, I deeply and completely accept myself.*

For Reminder Phrases try *"This emotional cause"* or *"I'm not even hungry."*

If you're still not able to come up with an event, memory, or connection, no problem. Just make something up. As I often say, a made-up example can work even better than an actual event or memory.

Tell yourself, *"If I had to imagine an event that could contribute to my weight problem, it would go something like this…"* Then use whatever event you create.

As soon as you have something, real or imaginary, that's connected in any way to your cravings or weight gain, create a short or long Setup Phrase around it and begin tapping.

These specific events are the building blocks underneath the bigger global issues. By dealing with them one at a time, they are easier to manage, and you can monitor your progress along the way. In addition, by going all the way to the foundation of the issue, you can start releasing these building blocks one by one until the global issue collapses.

Two points about this idea deserve special attention:

1. There can be hundreds or thousands of such specific events underlying a larger issue and thus, theoretically, addressing all of them can be a tedious process. Fortunately, you do not have to address every specific event to collapse the larger issue. You can usually do the job by collapsing somewhere between five and twenty of its table legs. This is because there is usually a commonality or "general theme" among those specific events. After EFT appropriately collapses a few of the table legs, a generalization effect occurs that serves to collapse the rest.

2. Remember that each specific event is likely to have an assortment of aspects, so address them separately and measure your progress on them one by one. Aspects can be the different emotions you felt during an event, the various emotional crescendos, or anything else that you would consider to be a "part" of your reaction to the event. The example given in Chapter One of the auto accident is a good illustration. Why? Because the event probably contains many aspects such as *the belief that it was all my fault; the smell of burning rubber; the sound of the crash; the smell of blood; the shock of the impact; my guilt at wrecking the car,* and so on. Each of those pieces is an aspect all by itself and should be addressed separately.

To be as thorough as possible with any specific event, use the Tell the Story Technique until you can tell the complete story without any emotional spikes.

* * *

In this insightful report by John Garrett, a woman taps through her tangled emotions toward her sister, thus freeing herself to lose weight. For your own practice, look for the Setup Phrases and identify which ones could be pursued as specific events and which ones represent global emotions.

Emotional Issues Had to Go First

by John R. Garrett

A client, I'll call her Tina, came to me frustrated by the lack of progress with her weight issue. She was morbidly obese and had been dieting and working out intensely for six weeks with nothing much to show for her efforts.

The day before she came to me, she experienced a confrontation with her older sister, Liz, who was a competitive body builder and personal trainer. She had asked Liz about what to do for sore knees from doing leg presses and got a lengthy lecture about her past eating habits. Liz chastised her for food choices as far back as when they were young children and criticized her for allowing her son to also become overweight. She prefaced these statements with, "I don't mean to hurt your feelings, but..."

My client was very hurt by Liz's unsolicited criticism and became defensive and angry at Liz's response. Liz also responded with anger and defensiveness, which created a huge, ugly confrontation.

By the time Tina expressed her feelings, she was ready to give up on the idea of ever being thin and fit, and she felt she just had to accept her sister's judgment. The fact that she could not remember what she had for breakfast while Liz claimed to remember what she had eaten as a child thirty-five years earlier made her incredibly self-conscious. She felt shame at being told to stop blaming genetics for her weight issues (they came from a long line of large people) and was hurt at being told that she and her son were fat simply because they ate too much.

My client was angry, but even more, she felt embarrassed and defeated. She carried intense guilt about her teenage son's weight issues and was horrified that he seemed to be following in her overweight footsteps. The confrontation with her sister confirmed her guilt, and it robbed her of energy and momentum to continue working out and following a diet program. In tears, she was ready to give up.

She decided to work with me not to resolve weight issues but to deal with the visions she had after the confrontation. She was so disturbed by these visions that she knew instinctively there was more going on than simple overeating.

Tina had thrown herself into her bed in tears after the confrontation with her sister. She dozed but didn't sleep. While in what she described as an Alpha or self-hypnotic state, she envisioned herself as an infant, with Liz, who was three years older, standing by her crib. Liz reached through the bars on the crib and pinched Tina hard on her arms and legs, intentionally making Tina cry. Her sense was that Liz was intensely jealous of the new baby and wanted to hurt her for disrupting her life and her relationship with their mother. Tina then had repeated visions of her sister covering her mouth and nose with her hand, trying to suffocate her. Several visions surfaced of Liz placing a pillow over Tina's face, which caused Tina to struggle with panic.

These visions startled and terrified Tina and were the main reason she decided to seek my help. Tina has studied hypnotherapy and understands that these visions may or may not be real events. She agrees that it doesn't matter to the mind whether they actually happened or are simply a creation of the psyche to explain her feelings about her sister. The fact was, they felt very real to her, and that was what mattered.

Tina shared that a few years earlier her mother had told her that Liz had always been jealous of her. Liz continues to have jealousy issues to this day. Tina's mother told her that she was very cute and outgoing as a child, while the older sister was sullen and shy. This outgoing, happy attitude caused Tina to get most of the attention of guests and family members and earned her the nickname Bubbles. Tina also had beautiful long white-blonde hair that caught the attention of almost everyone who saw her. Her older sister, on the other hand, had thin, wispy hair and was nearly bald until she was ten years old. When Tina was about five, her mother, exasperated by the older sister's jealousy, cut off Tina's beautiful hair, making it extremely short to match her sister's unattractive locks.

As they grew, Liz became obsessive about her body and her looks and was always dieting and exercising. Tina was involved in many other activities and paid little attention to her body until, as an older teen, she began gaining weight. As an adult, Tina admired and looked up to Liz and felt pride when cheering for her at her Liz's body building competitions. Tina, who was becoming more and more obese, also felt intense shame while attending these events, since they were so focused on looks and physique.

We began our EFT work with the statement:

Even though I am overweight, I deeply and completely love and accept myself.

In three rounds of tapping, her 0-to-10 intensity went from 10 to a 2. Tina yawned repeatedly during the tapping. We moved on.

Even though I have the memory of Liz pinching me...

Even though I have the memory of Liz smothering me with her hand...

Even though I have the memory of Liz smothering me with a pillow...

Even though Liz tried to kill me...

Even though my mother cut my hair to make Liz feel better about herself...

Even though Liz hates me...

Even though I hate Liz...

Even though I have to be diminished to make Liz feel okay...

Even though I have to be diminished or Liz will kill me...

Even though I have to stay fat to make Liz feel okay and not kill me...

Even though it is my fault that my son is fat...

The yawning continued, and Tina complained of being incredibly tired. She wanted to stop several times. However, we continued until there was no charge regarding thoughts of her sister.

Tina was obviously exhausted. She said she just couldn't do any more, then left and went straight to bed. She reported that she slept though the night and into the next day for a total of thirteen hours of sleep.

The next day, she was stunned to find herself feeling relaxed and content. She had little or no emotional reaction to thoughts of her sister and resumed her weight loss plan with optimism and vigor. She has agreed to tap daily for any discomfort that may arise from thoughts of her sister and to tap for accepting a new, thinner self. She has released a lifetime of fear and pain regarding her sister and now has the tools and confidence to achieve her weight-loss goals.

❖ ❖ ❖

In this next report, Dr. Carol Solomon demonstrates how a core issue can affect us in more ways than one. This is a great illustration of not only how our emotional issues can be connected but also how while addressing one issue we can gain valuable insight into another. If you are ever stuck on an issue, you might try addressing another one for a while and see if any insights start to appear.

EFT for Panic Attacks and Overeating

by Dr. Carol Solomon

For ten years, my client Margie had panic attacks approximately twice a month in the middle of the night. She would wake up startled and feel "very, very scared...panicked...not knowing what to do." She had tightness in her chest and difficulty breathing. She felt as though she was going to jump out of her skin.

Margie's mother was depressed, very emotional, and easily overwhelmed. Everything was "hard" for her, and whenever something was hard, it threw her off. She couldn't handle it and became even more depressed.

Margie grew up telling herself that nothing was going to be hard for her and that she wouldn't make a big deal out of anything. Growing up, everything had been an issue, so Margie vowed not to let anything get to her. She thought that if she let anything get to her, it meant she was "weak," like her mom.

Margie sought my help to learn EFT for weight loss and overeating. Her way of getting things done was to eat her way through it. "I eat three cookies, and then I do the laundry."

Margie thought her panic attacks were triggered by feeling overwhelmed by problems. Even though she wanted everything to be easy, she was easily flustered and "thrown off" by unexpected events. She would overeat during the day to cope, but whenever she felt "too emotional," she had a panic attack at night. It was a terrifying experience.

Margie used to have to take medication to get back to sleep. Now, she starts tapping right away and it relieves the panicky feeling.

Even though I feel really scared right now, I deeply and completely accept myself.

Even though I feel alone and scared…

Even though I don't think I'll get through this…

Even though it feels like the morning will never come…

Even though I feel weak…

Even though I vowed that nothing would ever get to me, and I would always be strong…

Even though it's important to be stronger than my mother…

Then Reminder Phrases as she tapped around the body:

Feeling scared.

Feeling alone.

Can't breathe.

Feeling overwhelmed.

I don't know what to do.

It feels like the morning will never come.

I don't think I'll get through this.

I'm afraid I'll fall apart.

Since I had taught Margie EFT for weight loss, she included weight-related statements in her second round. Notice the similarity between feeling out of control and panicky with her life and feeling out of control with her food and weight-loss issues.

Even though I feel like my eating is out of control, I deeply and completely accept myself.

Even though I'm feeling fat...

Even though I'm not strong enough to deal with my problems...

Even though I feel like I'll never be strong enough and I'll always be overweight...

Even though I shouldn't have any issues with my body...

Then around the body:

Feeling scared.

Feeling fat.

I can't control my eating.

I'm not strong enough.

It's not okay to be weak.

I have to be strong all the time.

I shouldn't be having this anxiety attack.

I feel like I'm not going to make it.

Margie views EFT as a "fool-proof method" to short-circuit her panic attacks. It only takes one or two rounds for her to stop the panic attack and get back to sleep. She has had only one attack in the past four months and has not needed any medication. She has also significantly reduced her overeating.

✻ ✻ ✻

Most of the Setup language above was directed at global material rather than specific events. However, if you take a look at the last set of Reminder Phrases, from "feeling scared" to "I feel like I'm not going to make it," can you see how each one of those phrases could point to earlier events? What memories does she have that relate to feeling scared, being too weak, or being out of control?

If your issue is stubborn or you're having trouble getting to the core, try asking yourself similar questions based on the information you have already discovered.

In this next report, Cathleen Campbell describes a successful businesswoman who gained weight when her work conditions changed.

Her Boss Was Making Her Fat

by Cathleen Campbell

Joan came to me to work on a crisis that was brought on by a change in her career. She was thrilled to discover that in dealing with this issue we could also help her finally reach her health and fitness goals, too!

Joan is a lovely woman, full of enthusiasm and joy. She's had her ups and downs in life, but mostly she's lived a pretty wonderful life. Her career has always been a point of pride for her. She has worked in the same field for over two decades, accumulating an excellent salary and a wide assortment of awards and accolades.

One of the special joys Joan relied upon was the affectionate and supportive relationship she's always had with management, especially her immediate superior. She loved working with Beth because they not only had a tremendous respect for each other but they also just simply enjoyed each other's company.

Joan was both excited for her friend and nervous for herself when Beth accepted a new position, leaving the department and Joan behind. Joan wasn't sure she would be able to recreate the same relationship she cherished with another boss.

Weeks went by filled with trepidation and confusion. And then the bomb dropped. The new department manager was a woman who had been transferred many times, and rumor had it that she was both ineffective and disliked. Joan was about to live her worst nightmare.

Before long she was questioning her very career, let alone her job and her abilities. She was miserable. Each day was a horror. She would take sick days and find other ways to be out of the office as much as possible. By the time Joan started to work with me the situation had become critical. She was fearing the loss of her job and feeling as though she had the weight of the world around her shoulders…and her waist and thighs, etc.

We spent the first session clearing the pain she felt this new manager had inflicted, using specific incidents and wording such as:

> *Even though my new boss is so mean to me, she yelled at me yesterday in front of the whole department and I felt so ashamed especially since she was right, I deeply and completely accept myself.*

> *Even though I'm nervous every time I talk to my new boss because she always seems so mad at me, I deeply and completely accept myself.*

> *Even though I not only don't have the connection I've always relied on with my new boss, but it's worse than that since she apparently doesn't like me at all, I deeply and completely accept myself.*

Since she hadn't known the new boss long, clearing this pain wasn't too difficult and Joan realized she was actually breathing easier and beginning to feel relaxed with this line of clearing. So we rolled up our sleeves and began to dismantle all the pain she had accumulated from the negative thoughts she'd been unable to stop thinking for months.

As we continued to clear through her personal criticisms, the ones she was aware of and the ones that she became conscious of as she continued to clear layer after layer, Joan began to sit up straighter and look more confidently assured. As if a light was slowly beginning to shine, dimly growing brighter with each layer lifted, Joan began to nod her head up and down. We finished a round and I asked her what she was nodding to, to which she replied, "I thought I was getting fat because of my age or the stress or my lack of exercise, but the truth is that I'm building a wall of protection around myself in every way I can!"

Joan's initial focus for her session work was her career, specifically clearing out the challenges with her new boss. She did this with very few tears and found it astonishingly easy. Now she was ready to face what was really getting her down: a load of added weight!

We began to tap for concepts such as:

Even though I have to protect myself from my boss in every way I can, which means I have to build myself up, I deeply and completely accept myself.

The look of relief on her face was a joy to behold, and her features began to appear calmer and younger. Joan left a bit exhausted but feeling terrific.

Over the next two weeks Joan kept in touch by email. Her final message said,

"I'm happy to report that I'm back to my usual habits—eating, drinking, exercise, sleeping, and performing at work. I feel happy and productive, and though my new boss is challenging, she's got some great ideas and we're started to get into a rhythm with each other. And the best news is that I've already dropped 10 pounds! It's melted off just as we said in session. My boss is not longer making me fat, but you know what? If she's right, she just might make my bank account a bit fatter!"

❊ ❊ ❊

The words of parents, teachers, coaches, partners, friends, and even total strangers can have a profound impact on our beliefs about ourselves. In this next report by Kathleen Sales, hurtful words held their sting for decades — until EFT removed their emotional impact. Her story is a great example of addressing a specific event for solid results.

Kathleen refers to the Sore Spot, which can be used in place of the Karate Chop point during the Setup Phrase, and the 9 Gamut Procedure, both of which are used in EFT's original Basic Recipe. They are not part of the EFT shortcut described in Chapter One, but they can be added at any time. See Appendix A for details.

"God, You're Fat!"

by Kathleen Sales

My client wanted to not only lose weight but also find a way to maintain that weight loss. She had tried many programs and had been successful at losing, but she always seemed to gain the weight back and then some.

I explained during our initial consultation that we could work on the issue of weight and maintenance but that we would also need to focus on emotional issues affecting her life since in most cases the issue of excess weight is not about the food at all. She agreed to the commitment and we were on our way.

I asked the typical questions about weight: *How long have you had a weight problem? When did you first recognize that you had a weight problem? Do others in your family struggle with weight?* And so on.

All of a sudden her face began to tense up as she spoke of her godmother, who had emotionally tortured her when she was young. Every weekend her family would make a trip to visit her godmother and godfather, and whenever no one was watching, Claire, her godmother, would exclaim, "God you're fat!" Keep in mind, this was said to a girl between the ages of six and seven, and it went on for three years.

The words echoing in her head brought great sadness and anger to the surface, so this is where we began. I asked her what her intensity rating was regarding this issue and she said, "Ohhhh, it's a 10 definitely!" While she massaged her Sore Spot, I had her close her eyes and repeat after me:

Even though I hear these cruel words, "God, you're fat," I deeply and completely love and accept myself.

Even though Claire's cruel words echo loudly, "God, you're fat," I deeply and completely accept myself and my body.

Even though I hear Claire's hurtful, mean, and cruel words, "God, you're fat," I completely love and accept myself anyway.

We then tapped on the EFT points using these Reminder Phrases:

> *God, you're fat!*
>
> *Those hateful cruel words, "God, you're fat."*
>
> *Claire's voice echoing, "God, you're fat."*
>
> *Those cruel hurtful words, "God, you're fat."*
>
> *God, you're fat!*
>
> *Claire's hateful, cruel voice saying, "God, you're fat."*
>
> *Claire's hurtful words, "God, you're fat."*
>
> *Those cruel, cruel words echoing inside of me, "God, you're fat."*

We also did the 9 Gamut Procedure, since this started at such a high intensity, followed by Setup Phrases to which we added the words *"this remaining…,"* and we did one last round of all the points while saying, *"I deeply and completely love and accept myself no matter what."*

I asked my client to remain with her eyes closed and go inside to see what was there. She felt a sense of calm. Her face had definitely relaxed, lightened up, and showed the results of the tapping. I then asked her to repeat the words, *"God you're fat!"* to see what, if anything, came up. She did and smiled. She said, "They're just words. They have no affect on me whatsoever. Claire is gone!"

At our next session I asked her to again repeat the words *"God you're fat!"* and absolutely nothing occurred. Just a smile and a shake of the head.

During the course of our work together, we found another person who needed to be "let go of," and when he surfaced my client said, "Oh goody, are we going to be able to make him disappear just like we did Claire?" We did, and it was another incredible result for EFT.

❊ ❊ ❊

Sneaking Up on the Core Issue

Sometimes the emotional reason for a craving or for overeating in general is an issue so overwhelming that it seems beyond help. It's the "Big One" that the person doesn't want to touch. It may be a major form of guilt that they don't want to face or a trauma they don't want to revisit. Whatever it is, they "don't want to go there" and often won't even mention it to their therapist for fear the therapist will try to drag them through it.

Often they learn to dull the pain or sweep it under the rug. But it seethes under the surface anyway, influencing their thoughts, their responses, and their everyday lives. It represents pain. It's like walking on thorns. They would rather retain their less-than-truly-functional lives than come face to face with this issue. Their lives will get better, they hope, if they just address life's minor irritations and leave the "Big One" alone.

Fortunately, we have a method with EFT whereby we can tip-toe up to the issue, circle around it, take the edge off, and gradually spiral in closer until that festering boil is skillfully lanced. All this with minimal pain. The concept is simple but it may take some practice before the practitioner can claim mastery.

It starts with a very general approach. I suggest asking the client simply say

The Big One

and then rank his or her 0-to-10 intensity regarding the mere mention of the issue. This is also an appropriate time to rank the intensity of other physical symptoms, such as a pounding heart, sweating, constricted throat, etc. We then use EFT in a general way to help take the edge off.

Even though I have discomfort about this issue, I deeply and completely accept myself.

Even though this thing seems too big for me...

Even though just thinking about it bothers me...

Even though my heart is pounding...

Even though [other physical symptoms]...

The details of the issue are ignored for now because the main purpose here is to minimize pain by taking the edge off. We are purposely sneaking up on the problem with gentleness as our goal. Do several rounds of EFT in this more general way until you see or experience signs of relaxation. That tell-tale "sigh" that I point out in our videotaped seminars is a good clue. Then say again...

The Big One

and re-rank the 0-to-10 intensities that this statement generates. Chances are the emotional responses will be lower and the physical symptoms will likely be down as well. I keep repeating this procedure until it seems appropriate to ask:

> *Is there any part of this issue that you could talk about comfortably?*

This simple procedure often opens the door, making it possible for the person to acknowledge or describe at least part of the issue. From there, it is simply a matter of getting more and more detailed. Take some of the edge off, get more detailed. Take some of the edge off, get more detailed. Take some of the edge off, get more detailed.

The client may experience some emotional discomfort in the process. After all, this *is* the "Big One." But, in my experience, it is much less than it might have been *and* this is probably the last time the person will have any such discomfort. Assuming our usual degree of success, they can now walk on velvet instead of thorns.

❊ ❊ ❊

In this next report, Carol Look draws on her extensive experience with weight loss and addiction to provide valuable insights into common emotional drivers. Please note that this article provides many "doors" that you can use to explore your own issues. Once you find a good "door," you will still benefit from identifying the underlying specific events and releasing them with EFT.

A Compulsive Overeating and Weight-Loss Protocol

by Carol Look

Diets don't work because they cause people to feel deprived, which triggers emotional and behavioral "rebellion." Sooner or later, after feeling deprived, you will overeat to compensate for the feeling of deprivation. This means that if you are using a diet to curb your cravings, it will most likely backfire on you.

Diets don't work because starvation mode causes hormonal imbalances and when the body perceives the danger of starvation, it "hoards" calories and fat for safety. This is why so many people complain of gaining weight or staying at a plateau when they are certain that their caloric intake is insubstantial. They are right. Their caloric intake isn't enough for their bodies, yet they start to plateau or gain weight again.

Diets don't work because they focus on the wrong target—food—instead of the underlying emotions that cause people to overeat in the first place. If you are targeting food as the problem, you miss the underlying cause of overeating, which is emotional stress connected to your past, present, or future.

The Present

The first section of my EFT weight-loss protocol targets your current behavior or symptom. Obviously there are many layers under the symptom, but to attack these first is an easy way to get started. Also, some of the layers don't begin to emerge until you target eating behavior.

The primary phrases that clients give to me about their "addiction" or weight problem include:

Even though I'm a food addict, I deeply and completely accept myself.

Even though I'm obsessed with food...

Even though I'm a sugar addict...

Even though I crave sweets at night...

Even though I have an enormous appetite... (We'll get to the underlying cause of this "appetite" later.)

Even though I'm a closet eater...

Even though I binge at night...

I ask clients to tap for themselves three times a day for whichever of the above phrases speak to them and their problem. I ask them to do it in the early morning and late evening when they are not in the middle of a struggle to NOT eat. Those who wait until they have a craving are less likely to complete the process, although one can do it then as well.

Two more interesting phrases that really seem to help some clients are:

Even though I have an urge to eat whenever I SMELL food..."

Even though I have a craving whenever I SEE food..."

These are very powerful anchors. Remember, advertising works.

Then I move on to the underlying feelings and anxieties that drive the behavior. Classic phrases that hit home with clients include:

Even though I eat when I'm bored...
Even though I eat when I'm angry...
Even though I eat when I'm lonely...
Even though I overeat to hurt myself...
Even though I eat to avoid my feelings...
Even though I use food to soothe myself...
Even though I overeat to hide myself...
Even though I binge because I think I'm worthless...
Even though I overeat because I don't love myself...

I recommend that you go fishing for whatever phrases ring true. If you are working with a client, you will usually see it in the person's face or you will recognize when it hits home.

Two other key points that I find essential pertain to guilt and self-hatred. These are not motivating factors for people who want to lose weight, so I help them drop the guilt about their eating disorder.

Even though I hate myself for overeating...
Even though I feel guilty when I overeat...
Even though I feel guilty about being overweight...

It's important to reduce these feelings so they don't backfire and cause even more overeating as a result of the anxiety. I use the tapping point on the index finger and say, *"I forgive myself for overeating…or eating when I'm not hungry…or eating when I'm angry… etc…."* This helps people forgive themselves for compulsive behavior that seems to be out of their control.

I worked for eight years at Freedom Institute with alcoholics, addicts, and their family members. The population termed ACOA deserves special mention. They are Adult Children of Alcoholics and were raised by one or more addicted parents or caregivers. "ACOAs" often suffer from free-floating guilt that would boggle your mind. They report feeling a gnawing sense of never being enough, never being a good enough child to help their parent stop drinking. *"If only I had been smart enough, good enough, clever enough, etc., mom would have stopped drinking for me."* Of course this isn't true, but eight-year-olds don't understand addiction. I always try to dig deep with clients who were raised with excessive dysfunction in order to get rid of the guilt and improve the chances of long-term success. Many ACOAs have sworn off alcohol because of their associations with an addicted parent but then turned to food as a more "acceptable" substance. Their underlying anxiety is often undiagnosed and untreated.

The Past

In this part of the treatment, I address basic self-esteem issues and incidents. I ask clients to write down or name three of the worst incidents that have hurt their self-esteem and tap for them. Often these incidents revolve around shame of their body or their early eating habits. I ask which is the loudest memory? The stickiest? The worst? I ask them to picture the first time they discovered food as a pacifier and address the underlying feelings that were going on at the time.

I also ask about their family's attitude about food, what the atmosphere was around the dinner table at home, etc. This often brings up new material, which I help them tap for.

Even though I'm anxious when I sit down to eat...

Even though I associate food with fighting...

Even though I associate food with my mother's love...

Even though I feel unsafe without food...

Even though I eat to feel better...

I ask clients to remember the sharpest criticism they heard around their body image, peer problems, etc. I have them tap for shame or whatever the strongest feelings are. This section can uncover upsetting times that may need more work. Go slowly and respectfully and you will make tremendous headway.

The Future

Next, I test clients to see how they would feel in the future if they couldn't binge with freedom. I ask them the following questions and tap for their reaction:

> *Picture yourself not being able to eat sweets in the evening. How do you feel?*

They often say anxious, angry, lonely, or irritable. We tap for the response.

> *Picture yourself as thin as you would like. What happens? How do you feel?*

This often brings up many answers. Sometimes they say they don't deserve it, or they feel anxious, or they don't feel safe anymore without their shield, etc. Sometimes they say they don't want other people to be envious of them or to comment on their body or appearance. We tap for whatever fears and feelings arise.

> *Picture yourself addressing the underlying feelings that trigger the eating behavior. How do you feel?*

They often feel anxious or just "resistant" to doing it and admit that they would rather suffer with the eating and weight problems. Tapping might go something like this:

> *Even though I'm afraid to face my childhood depression...*

> *Even though I'm afraid to deal with my rage at my father...*

Then I address specific sabotaging behaviors and ask them what their theories are about why they might sabotage their progress. I ask them to say the following statements out loud and tap for whichever ones cause a reaction.

It's not safe for me to lose weight.

It's not safe for others if I lose weight.

I don't feel supported by my family members.

I have often heard about clients who are offered chocolate cake just as they are making progress in their weight-loss efforts.

I don't deserve to be happy with my body.

I ask them to say out loud, *"I weigh 125 pounds"* (or whatever their goal weight is) and see what emotions come up. As in some sports performance Setup Phrases that are highly effective, I have them tap say,

Even though I have a block about weighing less than 140 pounds…

Even though I sabotage myself whenever I weigh less than 130 pounds…

Even if I never get over this eating disorder…

Even if I never lose weight…

These last two seem to help the inevitable feelings of desperation that most people with binge-eating habits struggle with. The clients often say they don't want to say these phrases because they're not true. But I urge them to say them anyway. It seems to reduce unconscious energy blocks about losing weight and stopping out-of-control behavior.

Obviously there are many more phrases and issues you can tap for. It all depends on your particular patterns. The most universal problems that get in the way seem to be shame, guilt, self-hatred, and anxiety.

Extras

Apparently, restrictive eating, chronic dieting, yo-yo weight gain and loss, and basic binge eating disturb the balance of our endocrine system and thus the metabolism. This is particularly frustrating to clients who have thought that occasional starving in between bingeing can help them lose weight. The metabolism reacts by holding onto every last morsel of food, expecting to be starved again in the near future. This often slows down progress in the beginning for some people, as their metabolisms rebel by slowing down. This is why you often hear people say they don't eat enough food or calories to gain weight, yet they gain anyway. I ask my clients to read up on insulin production, the basics of nutrition, and how stress affects the hormonal system.

I know there is a lot of bad press about low-carbohydrate diets out there, but talk to a carbohydrate or sugar addict or someone who is hypoglycemic, and they will tell you that it does matter what kinds of foods they eat and when. They find that breads and sugars trigger a compulsion to eat more breads and sugars. This makes sense when you consider the basic principles of addiction. Alcoholics in Alcoholics

Anonymous (A.A.) know that "One drink is too many, and a million isn't enough." This is how a sugar addict feels about sugar. It can be effective to tap for:

> *Even though I'm out of control…*
>
> *Even though I'm powerless over food…*

Asking the Right Questions

It is essential to focus on the correct "target" for your EFT tapping session. I ask my clients key questions to uncover the emotions that are driving them to overeat.

> *What are you really starving for?*

We know that once you have satisfied your bodily needs for food, the remaining "hunger" is not physiologically driven, but driven by underlying anxiety or emotional conflict. See if you can identify what you may be starving for in your life, other than food.

What comfort was missing from your childhood? Love, affection, warmth, attention? This "absence" may be why you're overeating as an adult.

> *When do you experience cravings?*

It's important to identify the times of day when you feel vulnerable to giving in to your food cravings. Once you know your "weak" spots, you can apply EFT before these times, heading off your cravings before it's too late.

You may use EFT before these time frames, or during them, when you are actually experiencing a craving.

If you didn't eat something, what emotion would you feel?

If you weren't using food as a form of anesthesia, what emotions might surface for you? Sometimes people don't know the answer to this question because they've never been "without" the food. They continually overeat so the emotions don't surface — that's the point of the behavior. See if you can guess or intuit what the emotion of conflict might be if you didn't satisfy the craving. Then you will have a specific target for EFT.

When you don't have "enough" food, what feelings are you aware of? Irritability? Frustration? Panic?

Guidelines for Your EFT Sessions

Set aside 10 minutes twice or three times a day to take care of yourself and address the feelings that cause you to crave unhealthy foods and overeat. Some people prefer putting aside a longer period of time once a day. It doesn't matter as long as you make the commitment to yourself.

Make sure you can accomplish this commitment. If you need to make the time shorter when you get started, do so.

I recommend using a special notebook to record your feelings and insights from the questions you have asked yourself and from the answers you get from your tapping mini-sessions with yourself. Make notes about what surfaces during each session, and return to emotional conflicts or patterns that don't feel completed during your tapping session.

Be clear about your targets. Do you know exactly what you are tapping on?

Make sure you are tapping on *specific emotions* ("the guilt about…" "my anger towards…" "my hurt as a result of…") rather than global problems, such as "I have low self-esteem."

Make sure you are totally *tuned in to your emotions*. Turn off the television and other distractions like radios, cell phones, and telephone answering machines, and make sure you have set aside a safe space for yourself.

Be clear about your "before and after" measurements on the 0-to-10 point intensity scale. If you have assessed how high the anxiety is before you start tapping, you have a good "before" measurement to compare after your tapping session. Record your results.

Write down any "AHAs" that you get from your EFT sessions. You may use these insights for later tapping sessions.

Good luck and be persistent. You will notice that you will soon begin to "forget" about eating binges and instead plan your food. And you will become engaged in activities other than secretive eating or food shopping. The weight will begin to come off as the underlying issues are addressed and the basics of symptomatic behavior are tapped away.

* * *

6

Eliminating Resistance

In any new project there are several ways in which we can interfere with our own progress. By becoming familiar with these ways, you can recognize them when they appear and then use EFT tapping to remove them.

By far the easiest way to reach a goal is with the cooperation of your subconscious mind. If there is agreement or congruence between what your conscious mind wants and what your subconscious mind has been programmed to accept as possible, everything is likely to flow smoothly toward the goal. But if there's disagreement or incongruence, the conscious mind doesn't have a chance. In that situation, the subconscious mind always wins. Somehow circumstances will conspire to prevent you from reaching your goal, and the conscious mind will probably never understand what happened or why. It will simply forget about the project or attribute your failure to bad luck or circumstances. It won't know that you yourself went out of your way to prevent your own success.

If you have ever made a New Year's resolution regarding your weight or physical fitness, you understand this syndrome all too well. Your conscious mind really wants to get your body into shape, and you may even start your new diet and exercise program with enthusiasm. But a week later, you're back on the sofa watching TV and eating potato chips.

Resistance to improving your life can show up in several forms. We have already discussed Psychological Reversal and tail-enders, both of which tend to operate behind the scenes and can be difficult to see. In this chapter, we'll look at more obvious, conscious forms of resistance and some easy ways to address them.

EFT can be effective even if you don't believe it will work and even if part of you doesn't want it to. Irene Mitchell, who learned EFT while recovering from a car accident, discovered this two years ago. She explains:

> In March, my daughter invited me to go on a cruise with her. She said that I had to lose at least ten pounds, though, as one gains a lot of weight on a week-long cruise. I had never practiced EFT for weight loss before, but I decided to try it. I kept at it and tapped every time I wanted to eat things I shouldn't. Sometimes I had to tap for the desire to tap.
>
> *Even though I don't want to tap about this weight problem because I really want to eat whatever I want...*
>
> After two months of tapping all the time and following a balanced diet, I dropped twenty-five pounds!! I have *never* had such a dramatic weight loss, ever!! Aside from the weight loss, there were

unexpected benefits. Naturally, I could get around better. I had less pain in my injured leg (which makes sense when you are lugging around less weight) and navigating in the shower was a lot easier. The best, though, was the fact that my sugar readings went so low that I had to go from twenty-five units of insulin each night to only five! My doctor is thrilled! So am I!

❊ ❊ ❊

Go to the health section of any major book store and you will find several books pointing the finger at sugar as the villain behind many of our physical ailments. Like tobacco and alcohol, sugar saps away our mental and physical functioning in insidious ways. Also like tobacco and alcohol, sugar can be an addictive substance. This contributes, of course, to a downward spiral wherein we crave more and more of that which is soaking up our vitality.

Helen Powell has faced a lifetime of sugar consumption and addiction, and she recently used tapping to clear herself of the problem. Please note the emphatic way in which she applied the process one evening. She says, *"I said it vehemently, I yelled it out, I listened to every word, I felt my resistance..."* This approach is often effective for stubborn issues. Here is Helen's story.

Emphatic Tapping for a Sugar Addiction
by Helen Powell

I too have a story to add to the countless amazing stories that abound in the world of EFT. Last

November I realized I simply *had to give up* the huge quantities of chocolate and ice cream that I was eating several times a week and sometimes daily. About ten years ago I began to notice a decline in my mental functioning and eyesight. I've read enough to know that it could be the sugar that was addling my mind but I just felt powerless before these strong cravings. Since then I began to experience more and more confusion, high levels of stress, difficulty in making decisions, mental fatigue, and more fears. Thank goodness, I don't have diabetes.

I took my first tapping course about four years ago. Since then I have used EFT with my clients and know how marvelously effective it can be. Even so, I wondered if tapping on this problem would *really* help *me.* The bottom line in truth was that I didn't want to tap away my fix. However, last summer and fall I did something so bizarre that I got scared. In October I did two brief tappings on *"I eat too much sugar"* but nothing happened, probably because my heart was not really in it. But maybe even that minimal tapping helped prepare the way because one November night, in desperation, I faced my strong reluctance to give up this bad behavior.

I started with the Karate Chop point, tapping on:

I don't want to stop eating all the ice cream and chocolate I eat, I just don't want to give it up, and I accept and forgive myself anyway.

I said it vehemently, I yelled it out, I listened to every word, I felt my resistance and accepted that this is just the way it is for now. I became fully engaged in the process. I did several rounds without bothering to measure my intensity on the 0-to-10 scale and then went to bed.

That was five months ago. Since that night, I have refused all desserts. What is interesting to me is when I look at all those "goodies" (are they really "good"?) something in me just holds back and refuses even though I can almost taste them. I have never felt deprived, not even for a moment. I've been to a couple of birthday parties where I surprisingly ate a piece of birthday cake without thinking, but I haven't accepted any other dessert without thinking as I was wont to do in the past. Maybe it was okay for me to do that because cake has never been my sweet of choice. I never felt guilty or frightened by these two iso-lated acts.

In January, I tested myself after looking longingly at a small package of jelly beans (no chocolate). I did buy it, and they did taste good, but I didn't really enjoy them. I don't consider any of those events lapses. And I am very happy to say I no longer feel as if I am losing my mind. The persistent haze that clouded my eyesight has disappeared as well. I feel much more confident and again really positive about myself and my future. Let me also add that I am seventy-seven years old looking back at a lifetime of chocolate and ice cream abuse.

❊ ❊ ❊

Here's a useful perspective by Angela Treat Lyon which points to emotional aspects that could underlie the stubbornness of some weight issues.

A Unique Perspective on Weight Loss

by Angela Treat Lyon

I've been working with an acupuncturist who uses Traditional Chinese Medicinal Herbs to help me drain the edema I have experienced since I was a young teenager. For years I had simply thought, "I'm fat. I'm overweight."

I had tried every last thing on the planet to resolve this weight imbalance and was at my last wit's end. I had dropped about thirty pounds already with what I thought was better eating and exercise. I had used EFT to overcome a chocolate/white sugar addiction—which worked like a dream the very first time, and I haven't even wanted chocolate since—and this is from someone who was practically weaned on chocolate. No more candy. What a relief!

Still, I needed to drop another twenty pounds before feeling close to my "natural" weight, where I'd feel light and strong and have energy without strain on my heart or muscles. I'd been carrying around the extra weight for so long that I had to buy bigger shoes, and I had been wearing men's extra-large shirts just to cover my large bottom. This all even after the great strides I had made since learning about EFT!

The acupuncturist told me that some of what I had been doing only exacerbated the problem. She said I was to avoid cold foods (no yogurt? no protein shakes?) because their damp condition made my whole body swell up. I love cold food. I was bummed. And she told me that my heart was weakened and very tired and that I needed to tone down my workouts to reduce my heart rate. I like to work out hard. Feels good. I was bummed again. And scared—my heart is *weak?* And *tired?*

I did a mini-rebellion and took the herbs she prescribed—but I ate the cold things anyway. And worked out just as hard.

And felt more tired, and more groggy, and more mentally inept and foggy. After a few days of this, I had to really ask myself, What am I doing? I'm paying to see her, yet I'm not doing what she recommends. So I asked myself why I would rebel against someone to whom I had gone for help. It was like saying, "No, no, don't help me down the ladder when my house is burning!" Duh!

So I tapped on:

Even though I hate it that she programmed me to think of my heart as weak and tired, I deeply and completely accept myself.

Even though I hate it that I have to cook more...

Even though I hate it that I can't eat my favorite foods and I hate it that someone is telling me what to do...

Even though she programmed me…

Even though it's all her fault…

Even though I think I have to cook more and it takes too much time…

Even though I have to eat food I really don't want…

Even though I have to do what she says…

…I deeply and completely love and accept myself, and I forgive myself and anyone else for my having gotten here in the first place.

I looked deeper. Thinking that my more-than-forty -year-old problem was her fault was absurd to the extreme— she wasn't even born when it started! I felt as if no matter what I did, it was wrong: that I broke out or got sleepy or became anxious or had some kind of unpleasant symptom no matter what I ate, and I'd rather not eat than go through all this. I'd rather die than hassle all this. I wondered—was I psychologically reversed to *living?*

So I tapped:

Even though it's not my fault…

Even though I want to blame someone else—anyone else—for my problems…

Even though I'd rather die than have to go through all this…

Even though I want to die, I don't want to be here…

Even though I'll never get it right…

Even though this is too much trouble…

Even though all food is bad for me…

Even though I can't eat anything or have any satisfaction…

…I deeply and completely love and accept myself.

I can't have any satisfaction? Whew! That hit deep. I looked at how I had made a career out of being creative and resourceful, and how I flew from one project to the next without giving myself room for congratulations or celebrating what I had just accomplished. Why on earth not?

So I tapped on:

Even though I am never satisfied…

Even though I have no real idea what that would feel like…

Even though I don't give myself the credit I deserve…

…I deeply and completely love and accept myself and everything I do or accomplish, and I choose to stop and congratulate myself and celebrate from now on, even if it's for only a moment, and I'll grow it more and more each time, because I deserve it.

I have been tapping on all those thing for four or five days.

Today I noticed a pronounced difference in my body. My pants are slipping off my hips (!!!) and I feel not just slimmer but more compact somehow. I can see it in the mirror, too.

I am now even more firmly convinced that it's not *only* food that goes in and out of our bodies, and it's not only what kind of or how much exercise we get. We also need to manage the energy in our body-mind system.

❊ ❊ ❊

When all else fails, persistence with EFT is usually the answer. Virginia Sabedra and her sister created a personal "EFT marathon" for weight loss while driving for an hour and a half in a car. The tapping led them from tail-ender to tail-ender on a journey that revealed many "behind the scenes" issues. Being overweight is rarely the problem in and of itself. Rather, it is often a *symptom* of other issues, many of them hidden. Personal EFT marathons may be a great way to bring them out.

Personal EFT Marathon

by Virginia Sabedra

Thought I'd share an experience I had a few weeks ago with EFT and my sister. My sister came to town to visit me. Since I had planned on taking a "fun" class in Oakland (which is ninety-eight miles from Sacramento, where I live), I asked my sister if she'd like to take the class as well. She jumped at the chance and on Saturday morning, we got up early, got in the car, and headed for Oakland.

As soon as we were on the freeway, I told my sister that I was concerned about some weight I was gaining and asked if she would like to work on this with me. She said she'd love to because this is an area she would like to work on as well.

She was a little familiar with EFT from my visit to her home a year ago. When I arrived at her house back then, she couldn't move her arm without pain. The first thing I asked her was, "What is it that you are shouldering?"

She laughed and then I guided her through EFT for about twenty minutes as her pain and stiffness melted away.

Anyway, back to the car and driving to Oakland. The drive is about one and a half hours long. We began EFT with the first thought about weight that popped into our minds, then that brought up another and another. Thoughts, beliefs, feeling, and ideas about weight and food abounded.

This belief that food is bad...

This belief that all I have to do is walk past a bakery and I gain weight...

This belief that the older we get the wider we get...

This fear that I'll never be slim and trim...

Tail-ender after tail-ender. We discovered that even the tail-enders have tail-enders.

After ninety minutes of tapping, laughter, sadness, surprises, and revelations, we arrived in Oakland and headed for our class. We wondered what the people in other cars passing us by had thought about us, two women in a car tapping their faces and upper bodies while mouthing words. We concluded that pretty soon tapping in cars will be a familiar sight. By the way, I was driving very carefully.

After our most excellent class we headed for San Francisco to have dinner. Then we headed home for another hour and a half of EFT and weight. You will not believe the "stuff" that came up with us both working on the same issue. When one of us came up with a super-meaningful tail-ender, we'd encourage one another with *"Ahhh, that's a good one,"* or *"Oooooh, that hits home for me,"* and so on as we just continued on and on, tapping, releasing and releasing and tapping, both of us throwing things into the pot, all the gunk about weight, food, women, traditions, holding on, getting your money's worth, etc. It was an amazing, eye-opening, revelation-inducing process about all the stuff we had stuffed ourselves with, as well as all the stuff that we allowed to be stuffed into us.

The next day, both my sister and I commented on how our San Francisco dinner had been different somehow. We thoroughly enjoyed our food, yet it was different. There was a freedom or lack of any thought about fat, fear, calories, and so on. Yet, we were observant of the food. It had a presence to it. We loved the food and how it was prepared. We ate differently in mind and body. I can't explain it well except to say that a shift of some sort had taken place.

The next day my sister's visit ended and she left. About four days later, I called my sister and asked if she had noticed anything about going to the bathroom. She stated that now that I had mentioned it, yes. She hasn't been constipated. I reported the same thing. Since our marathon, I have been regular. I mean nice and regular. I had always had a problem with this. My sister has always had a problem also. Yet, we both reported a cessation of constipation since our EFT marathon. Was it weight-related? In this case, I'd say so.

My sister and I are planning a second marathon on the same subject to see what else comes up and what results we will get, or where it will lead. We realize we have years upon years, and generations upon generations, of worn out, old, outdated beliefs, ideas, feelings, and notions to release.

I would say that during our marathon, we released months, perhaps years, worth of work on the subject of falseness, illusions, and negativity around weight and food, and other related subjects that automatically came up. In fact, I'm still processing to this day.

I have stopped gaining weight. Constipation-wise, I am *"nice and easy"* now. I spontaneously bless the food I eat. I ask and expect my body to process the food I eat and to let go of all that I don't need in a healthy way, and I am learning to appreciate myself in many ways.

I know that I am not "done" yet with my work. And, this is okay because as we work we continue to seek, explore, savor, experience, learn, appreciate, heal, and live.

This experience gave me the idea to conduct EFT marathons on various subjects. I conducted an EFT marathon on the subject of money in my office with a small group and it went very well. The collective consciousness of two or more people working and tapping on the same problem or subject has proven to be powerful.

※ ※ ※

7

Eating Disorders

I have been privileged to deliver keynote speeches at several conferences on eating disorders. Why do you suppose the organizers of those conferences asked an EFT expert to address their audiences? Most attendees are professionals: psychiatrists, nurses, doctors, psychotherapists, or social workers. What could EFT have to offer these very experienced professionals that they don't already know?

The reason for these invitations is that the conference organizers and the attendees are painfully aware of the link between emotions and eating. Thos suffering from bulimia don't purge for physical reasons; their behavior is usually driven by emotional pain. Likewise, binge eaters aren't packing food into their stomachs till they're stuffed becyase of physical hunger; they're propelled by emotional forces that override their body signals of satiation.

EFT can help those suffering from binge eating, anorexia nervosa, and bulimia to develop a healthy relationship with food.

Anorexia, a condition in which people starve themselves, can occur in men and women of any age, but it is most associated with adolescent girls. By itself, the term *anorexia* refers to a loss of appetite, while *anorexia nervosa* describes a psychological disorder.

Anorexia nervosa's most obvious symptom is extreme thinness, a body weight at least 15 percent below normal. Despite their thinness, those who suffer from anorexia nervosa have a distorted body image and see themselves as overweight. Three common ways in which they prevent weight gain are with excessive exercise, the use of laxatives, and by avoiding food.

A binge is any behavior indulged to excess, such as drinking, gambling, eating, or spending. Binge eating or bingeing refers to the practice of eating until one is beyond full. People who binge seldom notice what they are eating or how it tastes. This type of compulsive out-of-control eating is very different from the experience of appreciating, savoring, and enjoying one's food.

Bulimia, a binge-and-purge disorder, involves eating large amounts of food and then vomiting to remove it. An out-of-control appetite, feelings of anger and frustration, a history of fasting, the frequent use of enemas, purgative laxatives, or diuretics, and compulsive exercise may be additional factors. Often dentists are the first medical professionals to notice or diagnose bulimia because it harms tooth enamel and damages the esophagus. Bulimia also harms the stomach, can lead to dangerous metabolic imbalances, contributes to heart problems, and seriously interferes with the assimilation of nutrients, leading to malnutrition.

Anorexia, binge eating, and bulimia are rarely problems in and of themselves. They are usually *symptoms* of unresolved anger, guilt, fear, and other harmful emotions. Until a sufferer makes peace with the emotions that underlie the behavior, the symptoms continue.

This is why you don't hear a lot of success stories when it comes to treating these problems. Some people struggle long and hard and are able to control their behaviors with the help of dedicated professionals. EFT gives both patients and practitioners new tools to resolve the emotions that drive much of this self-harming behavior found in anorexia nervosa, bulimia, and binge eating disorder. There are many stories on the EFT Universe web site, written by both patients and practitioners, of breakthroughs with these conditions.

These are serious conditions and EFT should only be used concurrent with expert medical advice and support. Talk to your doctor or licensed mental health professional about your desire to use EFT. They may have heard of tapping, and they're very likely to encourage you in your use of a self-help technique that can help you change your behavior.

In this chapter, we will explore some individual cases related to eating disorders so you can see the complexity of emotional issues that we often find underneath them. You will also see how experienced EFT professionals have used their creativity and experience to work through them.

Like the other chapters in the book and the other books in this series, this information is not intended to represent EFT as a cure for an eating disorder or any other medical or psychological problem. What EFT is is a stress relief tool, and it works reliably for that purpose. Mental health and medical problems should always be adressed with a competent professional such as a doctor or psychotherapist, and this is even more true with a complex issue like anorexia or bulimia. By all means use EFT to support your current treatment program after consultation with your primary care provider, but don't let your enthusiasm for your initial results with EFT compromise your regular care. EFT works best in the context of a treatment program that offers you a matrix of techniques to support your health and well-being.

We'll use several cases to illustrate how EFT practitioners approach eating disorders. The first is by Karl Dawson, an EFT Master and developer of a form of EFT called Matrix Reimprinting. Here Karl walks us through the intricacies of a successful anorexia case. As you will see, there were many related aspects and core issues that had to be handled before the client, Joe, could resume eating normally.

Joe Resolves His Anorexia—and More

by Karl Dawson

At the time I was working with this client, there was very little on the EFT website regarding anorexia. I hope this article may help other practitioners tackle this issue. I did feel at the time that it was a borderline case and I was in danger of going "where I didn't belong." But, after speaking to Joe, I knew he had given up on the health care professionals. And as far as his parents were concerned, "the professionals" had given up on Joe. So I knew I had to try.

Joe's main problem was anorexia, having gone from 13 stone (182 pounds or 82.5 kilograms) to 8 stone (112 pounds or 51 kilograms) over a nine-month period, compounded by extreme anxiety, panic attacks, and self-harming behavior. Other issues that became apparent were an addiction to the artificial sweetener Aspartame, Attention Deficit Disorder, and feeling a loss of control in life.

Treatment consisted of eight two-hour sessions over a period of four weeks. Four of the sessions occurred in the final week of treatment, after Joe had been sent home from work because he passed out and was told to remain off work until his problems had been "dealt with."

In the first session I concentrated on gaining Joe's trust and mapping out some of the core issues that led a highly intelligent teenager from a good loving home to develop all of these problems. Joe insisted that his girlfriend sit in on this first session. This concerned me at first, but Emma was very helpful in encouraging Joe to work with me and happily tapped along, putting Joe at ease.

One of the first glaring issues was Joe's (and Emma's) addiction to Diet Coke, which is sweetened with Aspartame, a controversial calorie-free artificial sweetener which some regard as highly addictive neurotoxin that is added to many diet products. Joe consumed up to fifteen cans of Diet Coke a day in order to suppress his appetite and maintain a daily calorie intake below 500 calories.

We all tapped on this addiction issue with simple Setup Phrases:

Even though I have this addiction to Diet Coke, I deeply and completely accept myself.

Even though this Coke helps me suppress my appetite...

Even though I'm afraid I will eat more if I don't drink lots of Diet Coke...

Even though I'll feel hungry if I stop drinking lots of Diet Coke...

Very quickly Joe reported a loss of interest in Coke and his consumption dramatically decreased over the next few days to the occasional can and then to 0.

This first success was critical in my view because it gave a quick positive example of the effectiveness of EFT, giving Joe belief in the process, and it also got him off Diet Coke/Aspartame, which turned out to be one of the triggers behind his panic attacks.

The following events happened around the time of our first few sessions and illustrate Joe's frame of mind at the time.

Joe's parents had hidden the scales in order to stop him obsessing about his weight. Joe found the scales and weighed himself just as his dad entered the room. Seeing that his weight had gone up a few pounds, in conjunction with his dad observing this (In Joe's mind he was letting his parents down again in the only area of control he had in life), sent Joe into a suicidal panic. Joe disappeared for a few hours and returned with cuts and grazes to his hands and face. When I spoke with him later, he was in a desperate state and just wanted to give up. "I'm sick of trying," he said, "I don't care anymore."

I got a call early one Saturday morning from Joe's mother asking if I could come round. Something had happened that I never got to the bottom of, but when I met Joe at his house, he was in a highly distressed state. For fifteen minutes or so I just tapped through the EFT points, occasionally repeating, *"This emotion, this anxiety, this panic.'* Joe eventually calmed down but was not in the mood to carry on with a session.

After talking to his parents for five minutes, I went to check on Joe before leaving. Joe was having his hair cut by Emma and was perfectly calm. Joe recently told me that earlier that day he had been *"only a slight breeze away from ending up in front of a train."*

The dilemma was the eating issue. The last thing anorexics want to talk about or adjust is their food intake, but unless we consume at least 800 calories per day, the brain is starved of nutrition making any logical thinking difficult.

Joe had also grown wary of health professionals. He had already been treated by his General Practitioner, crisis team, psychologist, and anorexic specialists, all of whom he felt had abandoned him and let him down. Joe was under the impression that they were waiting for his weight to fall a little lower so they could hospitalize and force-feed him.

Knowing that staying away from the food issue was the only way forward, we talked about other things that were bothering him. I used EFTs favorite question:

If there was an event in your life you wish had never happened, what would it be?

It very quickly became apparent that a lot of Joe's problems had started around the age of six or seven at school. Until then he'd been a happy, carefree child. This I confirmed in a telephone conversation with his mother.

Joe's teacher that year was an elderly, old-school disciplinarian. From talking to Joe it was obvious he'd had some degree of Attention Deficit Disorder and/or Dyslexia, which had never been diagnosed. At the same time he was obviously very intelligent, leaving the teacher to draw the wrong conclusions.

In the first sessions Joe's memory of these events was vague to non-existent. In my subsequent talk with Joe's mother, she provided me with small amounts information, and we began to piece events together, sometimes just guessing what the teacher might have said in these situations.

The more we tapped, the more Joe remembered. Slowly at first, he started to recall memories which eventually flooded out, to the point were I had to write quickly to keep track on these issues to work on later.

I will let some of the Setup Phrases we used over the sessions tell the story of what had transpired between Joe and his teacher that year.

Even though I found it hard to concentrate…

Even though I found it hard to do math…

Even though I had trouble reading…

Even though I didn't pay attention to the teacher…

Even though Mrs. Smith said I was stupid…

Even though she said I was a little monster…

Even though I felt out of control…

Even though I would panic and shout out silly answers…

Even though nobody wanted to be my friend…

Even though I was different from the other kids…

Even tough I had to sit on my own away from other kids…

Even though the other kids laughed at me…

Even though I didn't fit in…

Even though my parents were called to school…

Even though the teacher told my parents I'm bad…

Even though my parents believed everything the teacher said…

Even though she said she tried to make me cry to get some emotion from me…

Even though my parents were angry with me for not trying…

Even though the harder I tried the worse I did…

Even though I let my parents down…

Even though I had terrible headaches…

Even though I gave up trying…

There were also many mental movies we had to work through, each one having several intense emotional highs and many aspects. A brief description of these were;

One day Joe found a note in his desk and on it was a list of things he had done wrong. His teacher said it had been left there by mistake, but Joe was terrified his parents would get to see it.

In her "infinite wisdom," the teacher thought tying Joe to his desk would be an excellent way to stop him fidgeting.

Joe had seen one of the other children dotting ink on his hands. He told a few of the other kids that the boy had measles. When the teacher heard Joe, she made a huge deal out of it and took the kid with the spots out of the class, telling them she was going to call the doctor and the boy's parents. Joe was left shocked and afraid of the consequences of his joke.

One day Joe and his brothers were being picked up from school. In a rush Joe's mum handed him a check and told him to hold it. Joe absent-mindedly put it in his pocket. His mother forgot she gave it to him and frantically looked for it for days. He did not remember having it until he found it in his pocket at school a few days later. He again felt he had let his parents down and was afraid to tell them, as they might think he had been bad again.

We also tapped using the Movie Technique on several recurrent nightmares he'd had at that age. He hated night-time, due to intense headaches and the fear of these nightmares.

In the main dream, he was alone inside his house and there was something dark and threatening trying to get inside the house and attack his sleeping family. (It struck me that these repeated dreams would also likely be trapped in his energy system. Would his subconscious have been able to differentiate between these nightmares and reality?)

It took a lot of tapping and reframing to bring the intensity of these dreams down. Again, at the start his memory was sketchy, but as we cleared one area, a new part of the dream would open up, and they were indeed scary.

Eventually Joe was able to go through the whole nightmare without emotion. He even gave his understanding on the dreams meaning. The exact understanding escapes me, but it had something to do with being petrified of having no control over events in his life and the effect his behavior had on his family.

Around this time in the EFT newsletter there was an article by Rebecca Marina describing the "Volcano Technique," in which clients are encouraged to feel and express their anger about situations that upset them. Because Joe often experienced extreme anger, we used this technique several times. As described in the article, anger can be a very empowering emotion. Giving clients license to really vent their anger — while tapping — helps to bring out and explode many other emotions. I found this method very powerful and have used it many times since.

Joe at 18 is a very polite, well-mannered young man. Even so, I think some of the language he used while we experimented with the volcano technique can be left to the imagination.

By our seventh session, Joe was ready to forgive his teacher, putting the way he was treated down to a misunderstanding on her part. He was also willing to forgive himself!

We did our last session over the phone. It was our fourth session that week, Joe had been very brave and had put a lot of effort into the sessions and was also doing a lot of tapping on his own. This was critical, especially with Joe. Self-empowerment of clients to me is one of the key elements and benefits of EFT.

It was our first and only telephone session. Something was on Joe's mind this evening, but he would not say exactly what it was. Joe had cleared an incredible amount of personal baggage, having undergone huge cognitive changes, in the process regaining a lot of self-respect and much more personal freedom.

In retrospect, I realize Joe was toying with the idea of seeing if he was capable of relinquishing his need to control his eating as his only form of control in life. Metaphorically I had a sense Joe was trying to reach the pivotal point of a seesaw. If he could find the faith to get past this point, his struggle would be an easy downhill ride—but he would have to let go and trust himself. We talked and tapped for an hour and he said he felt better. We set up an appointment for the next day.

Joe called me early the next morning, saying that he had decided to start eating again and that he wanted to cancel the appointment. Although obviously pleased, I was also concerned. That weekend I kept in contact with Joe's parents, and they confirmed he had started eating properly. Like me, they were cautiously optimistic.

Two weeks later Joe returned to work. He called me a few days before returning, saying he was slightly worried about facing the people at work, scared that the pressure and the attention he would get from them might be too much for him. He said he would tap on it.

A few days after he called to say he had gone to McDonald's with everyone from work to prove that he was okay now. But he gave the Diet Coke a miss.

I spoke with Joe this week for the first time in over four months. He now weighs 12 stone (168 pounds or 76 kilograms), is happy with his weight, and could never imagine so much as going on a diet. At the same time, he is worried he eats a little to much "crap food."

I wanted to ask him if it was okay to write this case study. He said, *"I believe your help and EFT saved my life. If it can help others, please write anything you want."* He said he is still tapping—when he needs it. At times he feels a little compulsive, such as when he feels under pressure, but EFT always helps.

He and Emma are saving up, as they want to travel round the world next year. He said he still thinks about what happened to him earlier that year and it scares him when he does. But now he says he feels 130 percent confident most of the time and can't believe how things got so out of control. "It seems like it happened to someone else," he says. He says he wishes he could get his mum and dad to do some tapping. *"It's about time they started dealing with some of their issues!"*

❊ ❊ ❊

We all overeat from time to time, especially at Thanksgiving and other holidays. In social situations that encourage overeating, it's hard to resist a second or third helping or another dessert. But when overeating occurs frequently and becomes a cause of shame or embarrassment, or when it becomes a darkly guarded secret, it moves from being an occasional indulgence to being a compulsion, a psychological disorder over which you have no control.

Binge eating has many emotional roots, many of which are often outside the person's conscious awareness. In this report, Dr. Carol Solomon shares her process with Carla's binge eating, then Carla shares her experience with food as a result of those sessions.

EFT Success for a Binge Eater

by Dr. Carol Solomon

To a binge eater, having one experience where you feel comfortable in your own skin is a success. Throwing away food because you didn't want it is a major breakthrough. A day without bingeing can feel like a miracle.

I have worked with Carla for four sessions. She had a traumatic childhood because of an abusive father. She associated food with survival, the only thing she could give herself for comfort. As a child, she promised herself that when she grew up, she could have whatever she wanted, whenever she wanted.

Carla already knew that EFT worked, since she used it to eliminate her need for her asthma inhaler. But she had not been able to stop binge eating. This problem can permeate everything you do. Carla had her life on hold. She wanted to build her business and start a new relationship, but everything felt too risky. The world was not a safe place.

First, we tapped on her belief that she can't have what she wants, so she substitutes food.

Then we tapped on her fear of promoting herself, of making mistakes, of the consequences of those mistakes, and her fear of being judged.

Finally, we tapped on one specific traumatic event, her sense of feeling unsafe in the world, and using food to ward off feelings of emptiness.

Here is Carla's letter to me:

Hi there Carol—Just wanted to update you that I seem to have had a breakthrough with our last session, although elements of earlier sessions are now accessible all at the same time!

Have not binged since Saturday's call without white knuckling (!!!!!) and I have in fact been having three regular (full of real food, but not grotesque quantities—just regular sized full of variety) meals!!!

For the first time in my *life* I threw chocolate away. On Monday night, I was given a chocolate at the end of Christmas meal with friends at a restaurant and I put it to my mouth to take a bite (habit—it was in my mouth before I thought about it) and it was too sweet and I was too full …and I held the last two-thirds of it in my fingers for over ten minutes as we were all saying goodbye, and I threw it in a bin *(threw it out)* on the way to my car!!!

I watched all the team at work pig out on candy-colored donuts at 9:30 a.m. and couldn't imagine anything worse so joined them without eating, without feeling like I cared what they thought (and they didn't!), and I was totally comfortable with it—*comfortable!*

I have re-tapped to Saturday's recording several times. I have also been tapping on more words around the language you have given me, such as, "That was then, this is now," which is really powerful. Lots of tapping with words coming to me easily around the promise I made to myself that was so strong through my childhood—my daily survival mantra—that when I grew up I could have whatever I wanted, whenever I wanted it. I really believed to my emotional core that food was the path, and only path, to my happiness.

It has "clicked" in me that actually that was then, and it was a little muddled, albeit well intentioned, and I can still honor my promise, just in a way that leads to my happiness by allowing me to be open to the things I want.

The tapping also seems to have kind of wired me up to comfortably connect with the new thought that salad and fish or salad and steak (*salad* and *meat* and *no dessert*—what is going on?) is actually the path to my happiness. I have always been able to physically feel better eating regular sized meals and easily digestible foods but my emotional drive to eat fast food fast, and lots of it, has always outweighed my physical discomfort every time.

These last few days feel profoundly different to me. My words to you are not sufficient for explaining right now—but they will give you an idea of how I feel so different!

I am nervous it won't last, so am tapping on that too. But that is the point, I am tapping (not refusing to tap), allowing myself to buy and prepare food, go to bed on time, and do the things that I want to do rather than assume it is too hard or scary and cop out and eat instead.

Today, I have the energy that comes from not being fueled only by junk food—amazing—so in itself, it is a relief.

It is unbelievably exciting—because I am not "trying." Today is Thursday, we spoke Saturday, and it has sort of just happened. It also feels like I have had a "click" in that I have been allowing myself to distract myself from the habit of constantly calculating the calorie restrictions needed for 40 kilos to come off in just a few weeks so that I magically get thin fast. I am feeling I can focus on just living and for three days have had no problem with taking time off from work or activity to have a proper meal. No Coca Cola in sight.

And on and on I could go…Much love and appreciation,

Carla

As practitioners, we have this driving need to help people, and it's easy to forget how much difference we can make in people's lives and in the world. When I receive letters like this from clients, I remember, and I am grateful for EFT and all of the wonderful practitioners who have dedicated their lives to helping others.

❖ ❖ ❖

After that letter from Carla, we might assume that four sessions was enough to tackle her binge eating. However, as Carol and Carla kept working, deeper issues continued to surface. The following is a second report of Carla's journey after eight more sessions. Listen in as Dr. Solomon helps discover, and resolve, several core issues.

Binge Eating Recovery

by Dr. Carol Solomon

My client, Carla, was aching to stop binge eating so that she could become more slender. As much as she wanted to lose weight, Carla viewed thin people as vulnerable, exposed, and weak. She somehow feared that she would "blow away in the wind" if she became thin. She thought she was being "shallow" in her beliefs about thin people, but it turned out to be much deeper than that and, as we worked, several core emotional issues emerged.

Even though I think thin people are weak, and I don't want to be like them, I love and accept myself completely.

Even though I'm afraid I'll blow away in the wind if I don't eat enough...

Even though I think thin people are exposed and vulnerable...

Even though I'm not sure what this means, or how I came to believe this...it feels threatening...like I might not even exist if I don't eat enough.

Reminder Phrases:

Thin people are weak.

Thin people are vulnerable.

Thin people are exposed.

They can't protect themselves.

I don't want to be like them.

I might blow away in the wind.

It doesn't feel safe to lose weight.

I don't know what this means, but it feels like some scary times I had in my past...like my very existence was threatened.

Through this sequence, Carla made some important connections. As a child, Carla's parents made her eat three meals per day, so that she wouldn't get "too thin," but restricted her from eating junk food.

Carla often felt deprived, so she would binge-eat in secret, and then eat her meals anyway, so her parents wouldn't suspect that she was bingeing. Whatever she was deprived of…that's what she craved. As an adult, Carla could not restrict herself to three regular meals without feeling deprived.

As a child, Carla had been abused. She "waited" to get through childhood, promising herself she could have and do whatever she wanted. As an adult, she refused to constrain her food choices and hated being told what to do. (She had a little five-year-old inside, who was stomping her feet and refusing to compromise.)

Even though I've been waiting my whole life to get through childhood, so I can have whatever I want and do whatever I want…

Even though I HATE being told what to do…no diet is going to tell me what to do…

Even though I don't like to wait…I want to have it right away…and I'm afraid it won't be enough…

Even though I refuse to be "without," even though it's costing me…

Reminder Phrases:

I don't like to wait.

I have to have it right now.

I might not get through the day.

It won't be enough.

I refuse to be without.

I WILL have what I want.

No one is going to tell me what to do.

You can't make me.

At this point, Carla began to describe her childhood abuse, in which she endured numerous instances of being hit herself and also witnessing her brother being hit by her father. Like many trauma victims, Carla would dissociate during the abuse. "I could disconnect my head off my shoulders," she recalled. "I could leave my body and be really still."

Carla knew that "being really still" was the key to her survival. As much as the abuse hurt, struggling or running would have made it worse. Carla's survival mode was to imagine that all of her weight was going down into her feet. Being "weighted down" would keep her from running and minimize the abuse. She even imagined herself wearing leaded boots that would anchor her.

Carla also believed that if she kept a layer of padding (extra weight) on her body, the abuse would be less painful. If the padding wasn't there, she would have no protection. As an adult, she still thought that the "padding" kept her safe. It didn't feel safe to lose weight.

Carla was incredibly relieved to make these connections. After addressing several of the specific abuse events from her childhood, her binge eating is greatly decreased, and she can now eat three healthy meals per day without feeling rebellious.

I have worked with Carla for twelve sessions. She was astounded by her progress using EFT compared to traditional therapy. Her question to me at the end of this session was, "How can I have accomplished more in twelve EFT sessions than I have spending thousands of dollars and hundreds of hours in traditional therapy?" That's EFT!

❊ ❊ ❊

While this next article by Dr. Solomon has a binge-eating focus, its concepts can be used for many kinds of success blocks. As she explains, "Since our work together, Johnna has gone from binge eating several times per month to zero binge eating for the past two months. Success! No reverting back to old patterns. This process, of course, can be repeated for other avenues of success."

Treating Self-sabotage Eliminates Binge Eating

by Dr. Carol Solomon

My client, Johnna, was incredibly capable, but she found herself continuously sabotaging her success. She would get close to her goal, whether it was weight loss or creative endeavors, and suddenly revert back to old behavior.

This was particularly obvious with her binge eating problem. Several times per month she would go "over the edge" and eat everything in sight. She made several attempts to overcome this problem but, alas, she reverted back every time.

It was as though a wet blanket was thrown on her drive toward her goal. Her inner critic would then show up, and she would have self-talk such as, "Who do you think you are?" Johnna did not believe that she was allowed to be successful in anything, binge-eating control included.

Johnna recognized her pattern of self-sabotage. There seemed to be some fear of success, but she couldn't identify the source of the problem. Keeping in mind her lack of success with binge eating, we started with some general EFT statements:

Even though success does not feel safe, I deeply and completely accept myself.

Even though success does not feel good, I deeply love and accept myself anyway.

Even though success feels threatening, I choose to love and accept myself completely.

Then we used some general Reminder Phrases to tap around the body:

Success doesn't feel safe.

Success doesn't feel good.

Success is threatening.

Part of me doesn't want to succeed.

Who do you think you are?

I'm not allowed to have it.

Part of me doesn't want to change.

It just doesn't feel right.

At this point, Johnna remembered that whenever she was successful, her parents would no longer help her. When she learned how to bake cookies, for example, her mother was happy and relieved. She would withdraw her support and turn that responsibility over to Johnna. It made Johnna feel alone, lonely, and overwhelmed, since she was saddled with more and more adult responsibilities.

She was always expected to handle these responsibilities. It was what her parents valued in her. But for Johnna, success meant losing contact with her parents, feeling alone and unsupported.

It was such a well-entrenched, unconscious pattern that as an adult, Johnna became anxious whenever she neared success. If she lost weight, she was afraid there wouldn't be any support and that others would expect more of her.

She routinely sabotaged her success in order to feel less anxious. Yet, she felt frustrated knowing that she was repeating the same vicious cycle over and over again. It was only during EFT sessions that these patterns became clear.

Once the patterns were clear, we identified some events from her past that were clearly causing these blocks to her success. Using more EFT, we resolved the emotional aspects of those events and Johnna soon started to feel the freedom.

Since our work together, Johnna has gone from binge eating several times per month to zero binge eating for the past two months. Success! No reverting back to old patterns. This process, of course, can be repeated for other avenues of success.

❋ ❋ ❋

Once again, Dr. Solomon shows us how effective EFT can be with overeating once you find the core issues.

Is It Safe to Drop Those Pounds?

by Dr. Carol Solomon

Sue was a binge eater who seemed to sabotage herself at every turn. She tried everything and lost weight many times, only to gain it back and more. She described her eating as being "like a runaway train." She ate to relieve stress. She ate to celebrate. She ate for every emotion she ever felt. And she felt like a failure.

Sue's mother always struggled with her weight and died of lung cancer at an early age. Right before she was diagnosed, she lost twenty pounds and looked great. She stopped dieting, but continued to lose weight. Sue recalled that her mother remarked, "Gee, I stopped dieting and I'm still losing weight." But the weight loss happened because she had cancer. She died soon afterwards.

Food was comforting, but Sue wanted to feel more in control, to stop bingeing, and to use food for nutrition, not as a drug. She lived alone and felt scared at night. She was afraid of dying, of going to sleep and not waking up. Every day, she ate sensibly.

Every night, she blew it. She found herself circling the pizza place, telling herself, "You're tired, you deserve it, you can start tomorrow." She was medicating herself to get to sleep.

Every time Sue started to lose weight, she got scared. She felt vulnerable. *It just didn't feel safe.* Food gave her that false sense of comfort because food and comfort were linked in her mind. Her grandmother fed her to comfort her. Her mother died when she lost weight. Part of her was afraid to lose weight, even though consciously, she desired it.

Strong associations can impact our behavior. In Sue's mind, food was associated with comfort and safety. Weight loss was associated with fear, loss and death. She was afraid that if she lost weight, something terrible would happen. Losing weight wasn't safe.

Binge eating is a coping behavior—a reaction to life's problems. It's easy to feel consumed by your emotions. Binge eaters often get into circular patterns of not sleeping well, overworking and feeling tired, and then being more vulnerable to bingeing.

Fears tend to surface at night, so Sue tapped at night whenever she felt afraid and/or felt the urge to binge. She tapped on her feelings about losing her mom, her fears of losing her co-workers, her fear of not waking up. Within three nights, she was able to feel more calm and relaxed and get more sleep, thus interrupting the vicious cycle. When her fears were resolved, there was no need to soothe herself with food. Within a week, she was no longer bingeing.

It's been a few months now and Sue's last note to me simply said, "I can't remember the last time I binged, and I've managed to lose ten pounds in the process."

* * *

Brazilian therapist Sonia Novinsky spends her time using EFT and affirmations to go straight for the emotional causes — and in the following bulimia case there are many of them, as you will see. The result of this emotional focus is a complete cessation of the client's symptoms.

You will note in Sonia's message that English is not her first language. Further, she had to write in a hurried state between appointments. Nonetheless, her conviction, caring, and skill come across quite clearly. Since writing this report, she has worked with at least five other clients with compulsive eating disorders, and all were treated successfully, with no recurring symptoms. Sonia's success is echoed by reports from other eating disorder professionals who have incorporated EFT into their treatment programs.

Bulimia in Brazil

by Sonia Novinsky

Shelly is my bulimic client. She is a personal trainer, thirty-four years old, married, with one child.

I worked with her for three months, once a week, from June to September, 1999. Then she came till

January once a month, only for checking, and the symptoms didn't came back.

Symptoms started in her early twenties (she got married at twenty-four). From menstruation phase (eleven years old) till age twenty-four, she wasn't allowed to date, go out, take a shower, or dress herself beautifully. All day in the bedroom, crying most of the time, feeling shame of being fat. Almost no memories of these years. Very severe depression after delivery of her child.

When she arrived she was taking Reductil (a weight-loss prescription drug) and two anti-depressants, Prozac and Tryptanol. When she left she was free from these drugs.

Symptoms: She ate compulsively, till no place was left in the stomach, mainly in the evening. Then she vomited or ran 10 to 30 km (6 to 19 miles) for sweating out all the calories.

Then she started eating again. Was obsessive about losing weight. Not fat at all. Three lipoaspiration surgeries in the belly and in the buttocks. In addition, compulsive shopping until bankrupt.

Using EFT and affirmations, I helped her work with the following family issues.

1. Her mother has been very sick since adolescence with a very rare kind of leprosy, no cure available. Very disagreeable spots in the skin. Shelly never felt permission to develop her own femininity. Guilty of being beautiful.

2. Grandmother living in the same house, taking care of Shelly's mother and the children. A very authoritarian person, violent, seducer and intrusive (including in sexual issues) — feelings of hate and guilt. The grandmother used to say that Shelly and her brother were responsible for the spots on their mother's body. Shelly yelled, "You are not my mother!" She felt guilty all the time and wore only male clothes.

3. Her father (a compulsive eater, maybe bulimic also, she thinks) felt in a trap, He didn't know the mother had this terrible leprosy before marriage. Violent conflicts at home all the time. She feels her father at the same time looks at her in a sensual way, and with contempt. Once she put her hand on his shoulder and he screamed, "I am not your boyfriend!" Very ambivalent situation. Feelings: Shame, guilt, and a lot of passion and rage.

   Whenever she felt better, thinner, or beautiful, and her father said a compliment, like, "You look beautiful today," this immediately triggered a deep tension and the compulsion to eat and throw up the food. And she start gaining weight again while feeling that food is in a bad place in the body and has to be thrown away in some way (through vomiting or aerobic activity). Feelings: Fear of being beautiful, fear of not being able to set limits, fear of becoming a whore.

4. Marriage issues: Limits issues with her husband and his family.

Results:

1. She is more comfortable when visiting her mother and father. No tension felt anymore.

2. No compulsion at all (0 on the 0-to-10 scale) for buying and eating food. No need to eliminate food from the body or to fast (she used before to fast some days to eliminate food).

3. She started wearing more feminine clothes. Shame and guilt = 0

4. She now can look in the mirror and love herself. Rage = 0

5. She is now setting limits and protecting herself from her husband's intrusive family. Being able to say, "I don't want you here today," for example.

6. More healthy relationship with job and career, attracting more stable clients.

❖ ❖ ❖

Six month later, Sonia sent in an update to this case. Her client Shelly still had no traces of bulimic symptoms, though she did develop other challenges with eating in response to new emotional stresses in her life.

Six month follow-up:

Shelly came today. Very interesting.

Shopping compulsion: Never more.

Bulimic reactions: Never more.

Job as personal trainer: Seven clients per day (earning money).

But something happened with her eating compulsion.

After our last session, I called asking for permission to tell her story to a magazine that invited me for an interview. She agreed immediately, but this phone call triggered a very anxious feeling: *"I can't deal with a success. I can't sustain a success, I prefer to leave forever, there is no durable success for me."*

After this she never tapped again and never called me back again. She just forgot me. It's a pattern. Whenever she has a success with someone or receives some public recognition, and she gave several examples, she leaves immediately and cuts the person off.

Then she was involved in a big stress in February because her husband went bankrupt, and she had some serious dental work. When this occurred, she gained 3 kilograms, or 7 pounds. She had been a constant 62 kilograms or 136 pounds since our treatment. Now she felt some compulsion but not a bulimic reaction. She is working very hard and has no time to indulge in a big compulsion!

I notice now a dissociation: A part of her wants to be 58–60 kilograms (127–132 pounds). Another part still can't sustain victory or success.

We will start another piece of treatment. She will pay me only if she maintains 58 kilograms (127 pounds) for a while.

Although some core issues remained untreated, including a critical one that allowed her to sabotage our connection and EFT, the bulk of our previous work is fine. She never threw up food anymore, never went to a mall to buy things on impulse, and she is very responsible in money issues, earning and sustaining her house practically alone now.

❉ ❉ ❉

Later Sonia submitted a final update. She described improvements in her marriage, a lack of triggering in response to her mother's demeaning comments, the ability to reframe negative events in a positive light, and noticeable improvements in various other parts of her life.

Final follow-up:

I think my work with Shelly just finished today. She is feeling great. I will see her next week for the last time. Today she told me some important feelings she had last week that give evidence she is okay:

1. She is dressing herself in a feminine way almost everyday. Previously she wore men's clothes because of her shame.

2. Someone said, *"How thin you are!"* And she liked this and did not feel the urge to eat compulsively after that.

3. Her mother said, *"The way you are using your hair is like whores use it!"* And she smiled and translated for herself, *"I am beautiful, my hair is beautiful, and I don't feel ashamed or guilty."*

4. She is in a wonderful moment with her husband. And when they were having sex and he passed his hands over her body, she felt appreciation for her weight, which is something really new for her.

5. Just before menstruation, when she normally succumbed to cravings, she realized she could eat a piece of chocolate and then stop immediately.

6. During the weekend (when she used to eat a lot), she now talks to herself as follows, *"I want to have the pleasure of being skinny, so I will not have the pleasure of eating a lot now. I can postpone my pleasure."* And she is playing with this new possibility in her life, to postpone pleasure sometimes. For example, she postponed the pleasure of reading a magazine she wanted to read as soon as she bought it, choosing instead to read it later while alone and in a peaceful moment, and so on.

7. She was alone Saturday night (a good moment for the compulsion) and she didn't feel any emptiness inside. She called some friends, drank a juice, watched a soap opera, and fell asleep. EFT has completely changed her life.

❊ ❊ ❊

Eating disorders such as bulimia are often complex and may take many sessions to resolve. Once in a while, however, we get a "one-session wonder" and major progress occurs within one hour. Such is the case in this report by Therese Baumgart. Note how Therese gets to the emotional drivers behind the disorder.

Two-Year Bulimia Problem
Improves in One Hour

by Therese Baumgart

Linda is a vibrant, athletic career woman and mother. Prior to her first appointment she told me on the phone that she had a food issue, but she was not specific. When she arrived in my office she said she had never told anybody before, but she had been bingeing and purging for two years. What began as a twice-a-month event had now increased to twice a week. As she related this problem, and through most of our session, Linda was very emotional. I used her information and often her exact wording to construct her EFT Setups and Reminder Phrases. Linda mirrored my tapping on herself as we worked together while saying:

Even though I feel ashamed and disgusted with myself, I deeply and completely accept myself.

This is a secret I never told anyone…

I'm so humiliated and embarrassed…

Bingeing and purging is my secret, and I'm so ashamed…

If they found out, they would say it's so disgusting…

They would say, Linda, how could you do that?

The worst thing in the world is for them to find out...

They would criticize, reject, and judge me harshly...

As Linda was getting ready to leave, she mentioned that she was most tempted to binge and purge in the afternoons. So for additional support during the two weeks between our first and second sessions, I recommended that every morning before starting her daily activities, Linda "set up the day" with EFT.

I also told Linda to follow her own thoughts and use them for her EFT Setups and statements.

I believe that part of Linda's rapid progress is due to her high motivation to help herself and her complete acceptance and enthusiasm for EFT. She started our first session extremely distressed and crying and ended the session with a huge confident smile, saying that she felt "wonderful."

Two weeks later, Linda reported that she had not had any bulimia episodes and had been faithful in doing her set-up-the-day phrases as well as tapping daily on whatever issues came up. She had even attended her family's Thanksgiving dinner and felt a little too full but had used EFT to handle the situation successfully.

During her second appointment we identified a core-issue incident from her childhood involving her mother, which echoed some of the emotions and thoughts around her bulimia. We used EFT to release these related core issues from 10 down to 0. Linda is now optimistic and confident about her continued success, and so am I.

After her first session, Linda wrote, "As I reflect on the last one and a half weeks since we met, the overall sense I have is that the torment is gone from my relationship with food. Before I came to see you and had my first EFT session, I had definite feelings of inadequacy, hopelessness, and helplessness about bingeing and my weight. I did not realize the amount of shame I felt about my actions in the area of bingeing.

"I have to say for the first time," she concluded, "that I feel like I have a healthy home inside myself, a place I can go, through tapping, that soothes, comforts, and cares for me and my feelings. I hear the torment and I 'go home' to the comfort and compassion of the tapping session. It is truly a relief and grace for me. I look forward to our next session."

❈ ❈ ❈

In this next report from Aileen Nobles, one professionally applied session brought relief to a client who went from bingeing and purging twice a day to zero occurrences in the following six weeks.

A Bulimia "One-Session Wonder"

by Aileen Nobles

About a month ago a client came to me with major anxiety issues. She had reverted back to a bulimic pattern that she has had on and off since she was a teen.

She's in her late thirties now. She fully understood the dangers of this behavior but had been eating and purging twice a day for the last four months.

She was very clear as to when it first started. Her mother had been at a birthday party with her and she had eaten too much cake and didn't feel so well. Her mother told her that if she could make herself throw up she would feel better. She did...and, indeed, she felt better!

She also said that she was teased at school about her body, yet if she looked at a photo of herself at school, she saw that she wasn't fat.

We did a basic round on:

Even though my mother suggested I throw up if I've eaten too much, I can still completely accept myself.

Even though I'm trying to throw up all of my anxiety, fear, and ugly feelings about myself, It's okay. I can still completely accept myself.

My mother didn't always suggest the best things for me, and throwing up after eating is one of them.

I chose to use "is" instead of "was" to bring these events into present time. We did another round on:

My mother drank too much and didn't feel good about herself so she put a lot of pressure on me to look and perform a certain way.

The client had been a child actor.

I then suggested that she relax and imagine all of the negative images that came from her mother and the children at school. We started tapping on her issues of anxiety and fear and brought those levels way down.

We went back to:

Even though I can't get rid of my fear and anxiety by throwing it up, I deeply and completely accept myself.

Even though it would be much better if I don't overeat in the first place...

We went on to issues of not liking the way she looks. I asked her to tell me what she disliked and liked about her appearance. She focused on disliking her legs, thighs, and behind. She suddenly remembered very vividly being called "fat ass" in school. It still triggered a strong reaction as she thought about it. We tapped on:

Even though I have a fat ass, I don't need to throw up.

I threw in a reframe about the size of Serena Williams' rear end and how it was revered by thousands. (My client actually has a nice fairly small curved rear end.)

It's been six weeks now and, so far, she has had no desire to binge. Please recall that, before EFT, she was bingeing and purging twice a day. She taps on herself for the anxiety and fear. I just love it when EFT works this well.

✳ ✳ ✳

8

Your Plan for Long-Term
Weight Loss with EFT

As you now know, EFT is phenomenally effective for weight loss. Studies show that, as you use EFT, you can not only lose weight, but keep it off permanently (Stapleton, Sheldon, & Porter, 2011; Church & Wilde, 2013). You've now read the stories of dozens of people who've had this experience, and you've started to use EFT yourself. You've probably already had insights and breakthroughs that have changed your relationship to food, and you're likely to have more as you persist with EFT.

You're serious about weight loss. What should you do each day, each meal, each week, each year in order to apply EFT most effectively to lose weight and maintain your gains?

This final chapter of the book gives you a Tapping Plan for Weight Loss. It provides you with recommendations about what to do on a daily basis, and how to tap long term. If you follow this plan, you will remove most of the emotional associations you have with food. I summarize the plan below. You'll also find an abbreviated form of these recommendations on a single page at the end of the book. Make copies of that plan and pin it up on your refrigerator. Tape it to your bathroom mirror, and keep a copy in your purse or wallet. These are practices to remind yourself of daily till they become second nature.

Continuous Tapping

One of the phrases I use is "continuous tapping." This is the easiest way of applying EFT that you can imagine. In most cases it dispenses with the SUD score, the Setup Statement, and the other parts of EFT's Basic Recipe. You simply tap on each point, then move on to the next. When you get to the last point, you start again with the Karate Chop point. When doing continuous tapping, always tap the Karate Chop as the first point. Then tap the eyebrow point, the side of the eye point, and so on till you get to the underarm point. Then tap the Karate Chop point again as you start another round of EFT. For instance, I recommend continuous tapping while you eat a food you crave. The way you apply this recommendation is simply to sit down and eat some of that food with one hand, while tapping continuously with the other hand. That's all you have to do, so it couldn't be easier. You don't have to remember the right words, or any words at all. You just have your experience with the food while you tap continuously throughout. When compared with any other weight loss intervention, you'll find nothing easier. Yet this one act of soothing your emotions while tapping when combined with eating can make profound changes in your relationship with food.

The Importance of Planning

I've divided the Tapping Plan for Weight Loss into six parts. The first is things you do each morning when you wake up. This is an important step. By setting your intentions for the day, and tapping on them, you remind your mind, body, and heart what you plan to do during the coming day. You might not be able to carry out all those intentions. Life happens, and it rarely goes according to plan. There's a saying by General Norman Schwartzkopf, "No battle plan survives first contact with the enemy." But that doesn't mean you shouldn't plan. A plan gives concrete form to your intentions, and provides you with a general outline of what you expect even if every detail doesn't materialize. General Dwight Eisenhower said, "Plans are futile. Planning is essential." So tap and plan your day even though you'll need to respond with flexibility to unforeseen events.

Incorporating Tapping into Eating

As you follow the plan given here, you'll find yourself tapping regularly throughout each day. As I'm writing this, I'm looking at a beautiful view. I'm visiting my family in Jacksonville, Florida, and my hotel suite looks out over the St. John's River and downtown Jacksonville. I'm sitting on a balcony and the sun is rising. The boats in the marina across the river are catching the sun's rays, and the water is shimmering. I know there's a breakfast buffet downstairs in the hotel lobby, and my tummy is rumbling. I'm looking forward to being able to choose the healthiest foods I know support my weight loss goals.

There's just one negative trigger. My balcony is located above a ventilation duct for the hotel kitchen, and smells are wafting upwards. The predominant one is syrup. Now I don't usually crave syrup, because the fake rubbish maple syrup substitute they serve at hotel buffets is way too sweet and packed with artificial ingredients. But this morning the smell is reminding me of how hungry I am, and how long it was since last night's meal with my family.

The scent of that syrup evoked a craving of about a 9 to begin with. I was contemplating abandoning my writing and going to eat earlier than I planned. After three rounds of continuous tapping, the smell is simply pleasant, about a 2, and I continue with my writing.

I've invited my whole family over to the suite this evening for food and wine. While I tap, I imagine how the evening will go. I expect to enjoy the company, and also eat moderately. I'll drink some wine, but then switch to soda water before I drink too much. As I tap, I remember that I need to buy some soda water when I pick up the food.

You'll find yourself setting yourself up for success each day as you do similar tapping. Will you always stick with your plan? You might binge, or forget, and eat or drink far more than you planned. No problem. Just use EFT's wonderful phrase "I deeply and completely accept myself" and go right back to the plan the next day.

If you can't tap, for instance, when eating a meal with a client, then tap mentally. If you're following the recommendation to tap when sitting down to a meal but before eating it, simply imagine tapping each point in your mind before you begin eating. You won't look weird, your client won't know, and you'll still keep your commitment to sticking with your weight loss plan.

Tapping Plan for Weight Loss (Extended Version)

Morning:

Review in detail your eating plan for the day, meal by meal, snack by snack, while tapping continuously.

Tap continuously while you weigh yourself.

Look at your face in the mirror and say "I deeply and completely accept myself" slowly five times while tapping and breathing deeply.

Review in detail your exercise plan for the day while tapping continuously.

Daily:

Tap immediately after any negative interaction with another person. Replay the interaction in your mind while tapping continuously till your SUD level is 2 or less.

Whenever you recall any negative past event around food or body image, do three rounds of EFT.

Whenever you catch yourself in a piece of negative self-talk, tap on that negative phrase till it has a SUD score of 2 or less.

Tap continuously whenever you see or smell a food that triggers a craving.

While exercising, tap mentally, or physically if possible.

Before Each Meal:

After you sit down to eat a meal, before starting, tune in to your body, and notice any sensations that arise. Also contemplate the meal with its sights and smells. Complete three rounds of tapping before taking the first bite.

Before eating a food you crave, sit with that food, and tap continuously through five rounds of EFT while focusing on how the food looks and smells.

During Each Meal:

Put your utensils down after the first three bites of food, and complete another round of tapping.

While eating with one hand a food you crave, tap continuously with your other hand.

Tap when theres's some food left on your plate after a meal and you aren't sure whether or not to eat it.

When you're finished eating, look at your plate and tap three rounds.

When You Slip:

Tap continuously while repeating the phrase, "I forgive myself. Even though I slipped, I deeply and completely accept myself."

Notice any body sensations that arise when you think about your slip. Tap till they have a SUD score of 2 or less.

Notice any self-talk that comes up, such as "There I go again," or similar negative phrases. Notice your body sensations associated with the phrase, and tap till the SUD score is 2 or less.

Evening:

Review what you ate today and your experiences with tapping, while tapping continuously.

If during the course of the day you recalled any negative events from earlier in your life, tap on them till they have a SUD score or 2 or less.

While tapping continuously, say, "I fall asleep quickly and easily, and sleep soundly through the night. I lose weight while I sleep. I wake up in the morning feeling completely refreshed."

Next Steps

Tapping reinforces everything else you do to support your health. This book has shown you exactly what those people who are successful at weight loss do. It's offered you dozens of tips from experts. It's shown you how to apply EFT to cultivate healthy weight loss behaviors. It's demonstrated over and over again that success is possible and even easy, no matter how many times you've failed in the past. Please continue taking action till you've met and maintained your weight goals. Here are some additional ways you can support yourself in your weight loss journey. I strongly recommend you take these seven steps:

1. The Personal Peace Procedure

The first is to use what EFT calls the Personal Peace Procedure. The Personal Peace Procedure basically recommends that you buy a blank personal journal and write down the key emotionally traumatic events that have happened in your life. You'll find full instructions for this in our free tutorial on the EFT Universe website, and in Chapter 1 of this book.

You may have had hundreds of events throughout your life that bothered you, upset you, or made you angry. Writing them all down in a journal and looking at them isn't always fun. If there are hundreds of events in your childhood, healing them all might seem like an overwhelming task.

Yet if you then just tap on three of them a day, and reduce your number from a 5, 7, or 10 down to a 0, 1, or 2, you can make fast progress on erasing all that emotional trauma. Tapping on just three a day, in a year you can tap on 1,000 different events. That cleans up a huge chunk of your childhood. I recommend you purchase a personal journal and follow the Personal Peace Procedure.

2. The 9 Gamut Procedure

The second thing I recommend you do is familiarize yourself with EFT's 9 Gamut Procedure. It's described in *The EFT Manual* (Church, 2013). There's also a description of the 9 Gamut Procedure, along with a free Tap-Along Video, on the EFT Universe website. The 9 Gamut Procedure is very useful as an add-on if the Basic Recipe we taught you in this program isn't working for a particular problem, or isn't working fast enough.

3. EFT Workshops

I also strongly recommend that you take an EFT workshop. The EFT workshops have been designed based on watching thousands of people learn EFT, seeing precisely how they assimilate the information, and then training them in expert use of EFT.

We've analyzed the steps by which people learn EFT and apply it most successfully; each level of the program is divided into eight learning modules. In those modules, you learn the basics of EFT step-by-step. You discover how to apply it effectively to many different situations. Certified EFT Universe instructors teach EFT workshops all over the world; you can enroll in one near you through the web link. Workshops are the way to unlock the full power of EFT.

4. Search for Stories Like Yours

EFT Universe contains some 10,000 stories in over a dozen different languages. You will likely find stories written by people who have faced the same situations you have, and have used EFT successfully. From their stories, you can glean tips, techniques, and ways of using EFT that will help you on your journey. It's absolutely free, easy to do, and easily searchable.

There are three different ways you can unlock the riches of EFT Universe. The first is to use the search engine on the EFT Universe website. There's also an Advanced Search option.

Second, you can find a quick-start list of the most common problems on the Case Histories page.

Finally, on the home page of www.EFTUniverse. com, notice the drop-down menu titled "Choose a Topic." Here you'll find stories grouped by subject.

Even though the website is vast, it's so intuitively organized that you'll quickly find what you need. Hundreds of thousands of people visit EFT Universe each month and find solutions to their problems. You don't need to feel alone facing your challenges, and you'll find like-minded friends at EFT Universe.

5. Tapping Circles

I recommend you join a Tapping Circle. These are groups of people that get together to work with each other on their issues. They may be online groups, or they may meet in person. You can find tapping circles on the "Volunteering" page on the EFT Universe.

6. Discussion Groups

You can also ask questions in the EFT Universe Discussion Groups. We have discussion groups covering many different common topics, from PTSD to Addictions to Children to Weight Loss to Pain. Go there, ask your questions and get advice from people who have traveled the same journey that lies ahead of you.

7. Certified Practitioners

I strongly recommend booking a session with one of our EFT Universe Certified Practitioners. These practitioners go a through rigorous training in Clinical EFT. If they're listed on our site, we have confidence that they can help you. You can search the practitioner database by name, state, and specialty to find the perfect practitioner for your needs. Many of them offer a free introductory session, so you can interview a number of practitioners to find a good fit.

My final word of advice is to tap immediately. When you're in any kind of an emotional jam or physical need, start tapping right away. Don't worry about finding the right words to say, or even whether you're tapping the correct points. Doing EFT is more important than doing EFT perfectly. It's hard to mess up EFT. Start tapping. You'll find that it has a calming, soothing effect on your body, even if you "do it wrong."

Once you've calmed yourself, you can check the manual, search the site, find a practitioner, or take other steps toward solving your problem. Don't delay tapping till you have one of those resources at your disposal. When in doubt, tap! You'll find yourself better equipped to deal with whatever stress faces you.

I urge you to love yourself enough to learn EFT, memorize EFT, and equip yourself with EFT. You'll then find that whatever the stress, strain, or emergency, you have a potent tool at your fingertips. EFT will help you deal with the problem, get through those stresses, and come out on the other side. You'll progress much more quickly, feel much better, and attain a much higher level of health and vitality.

References

Church, D. (2013). *The EFT Manual* (3rd ed.). Santa Rosa, CA: Energy Psychology Press.

Church, D. & Wilde, N. (2013, May). Emotional eating and weight loss following Skinny Genes, a six week online program. Reported at the annual conference of the Association for Comprehensive Energy Psychology (ACEP), Reston, VA.

Stapleton, P. B., Sheldon, T., & Porter, B. (2012). Clinical benefits of Emotional Freedom Techniques on food cravings at 12-months follow-up: A randomized controlled trial. *Energy Psychology: Theory, Research, and Treatment, 4*(1), 1–12.

EFT Glossary

The following terms have specific meanings in EFT. They are referred to in some of the reports included here and are often mentioned in EFT reports.

Acupoints. Acupuncture points that are sensitive points along the body's meridians. Acupoints can be stimulated by acupuncture needles or, in acupressure, by massage or tapping. EFT is an acupressure tapping technique.

Art of Delivery. The sophisticated presentation of EFT that uses imagination, intuition, and humor to quickly discover and treat the underlying causes of pain and other problems. The art of delivery goes far beyond basic EFT.

Aspects. "Issues within issues," or different facets or pieces of a problem that are related but separate. When new aspects appear, EFT can seem to stop working. In truth, the original EFT treatment continues to work while the new aspect triggers a new set of symptoms. In some cases, many aspects of a situation or problem each require their own EFT treatment. In others, only a few do.

Basic Recipe (also known as Mechanical EFT). EFT's basic protocol, which consists of tapping on the Karate Chop point or Sore Spot while saying three times, "Even though I have this ___[problem]___, I fully and complete accept myself" (Setup Phrase), followed by three rounds of tapping the Sequence of EFT acupoints in order, with an appropriate Reminder Phrase. See also Full Basic Recipe.

Borrowing Benefits. When you tap with or on behalf of another person, your own situation improves, even though you aren't tapping for your own situation. This happens in one-on-one sessions, in groups, and when you perform surrogate or proxy tapping. The more you tap for others, the more your own life improves.

Chasing the Pain. After applying EFT, physical discomforts can move to other locations and/or change in intensity or quality. A headache described as a sharp pain behind the eyes at an intensity of 8 might shift to a dull throb at the back of the head at an intensity of 7 (or 9, or 3, or any other intensity level). Moving pain is an indication that EFT is working. Keep "chasing the pain" with EFT and it will usually go to 0 or some low number. In the process, emotional issues behind the discomforts are often successfully treated.

Chi. Vital energy that flows through and around every living being. Chi is said to regulate spiritual, emotional, mental, and physical balance and to be influenced by *yin* (the receptive, feminine force) and *yang* (the active masculine force). These forces, which are complementary opposites, are in constant motion. When yin and yang are balanced, they work together with the natural flow of chi to help the body achieve and maintain health. Chi moves through the body along invisible pathways, or channels, called meridians. Traditional Chinese medicine identifies twenty meridians through which chi flows or circulates to all parts of the body. Acupoints along the meridians can be stimulated to improve the flow of chi and, in EFT, to resolve emotional issues.

Choices Method. Dr. Patricia Carrington's method for inserting positive statements and solutions into Setup and Reminder Phrases.

Core Issues. Deep, important underlying emotional imbalances, usually created in response to traumatic events. A core issue is truly the crux of the problem, its root or heart. Core issues are not always obvious but careful detective work can often uncover them and, once discovered, they can be broken down into specific events and handled routinely with EFT.

Full Basic Recipe. A four-step treatment consisting of Setup phrase, Sequence (tapping on acupoints in order), 9-Gamut Procedure, and Sequence. This was the original EFT protocol.

Generalization Effect. When related issues are neutralized with EFT, they often take with them issues that are related in the person's mind. In this way, several issues can be resolved even though only one is directly treated.

Global. Though the term "global" usually refers to something universal or experienced worldwide, in EFT it refers to problems stated in vague and nonspecific terms, especially in Setup Phrases.

Intensity Meter. The 0-to-10 scale that measures pain, discomfort, anger, frustration, and every other physical or emotional symptom. Intensity can also be indicated with gestures, such as hands held close together (small discomfort) or wide apart (large discomfort).

Mechanical EFT. See Basic Recipe.

Meridians. Invisible channels or pathways through which energy *(chi)* flows in the body. The eight primary meridians pass through five pairs of vital organs, and twelve secondary meridians network to the extremities. The basic premise of EFT is that the cause of every negative emotion and most physical symptoms is a block or disruption in the flow of chi along one or more of the meridians.

Movie Technique, or Watch the Movie Technique. In this process, you review in your mind, as though it were a movie, a bothersome specific event. When intensity comes up, stop and tap on that intensity. When the intensity subsides, continue in your mind with the story. This method has been a mainstay in the toolbox of many EFT practitioners. It may be the most-used EFT technique.

Personal Peace Procedure. An exercise in which you clear problems and release core issues by writing down, as quickly as possible, as many bothersome events from your life that you can remember. Try for at least fifty, or a hundred. Give each event a title, as though it is a book or movie. When the list is complete, begin tapping on the largest issues. Eliminating at least one uncomfortable memory per day (a very conservative schedule) removes at least ninety unhappy events in three months. If you work through two or three per day, it's 180 or 270.

Reminder Phrase. A word, phrase, or sentence that helps the mind focus on the problem being treated. It is used in combination with acupoint tapping.

Setup Phrase, or Setup. An opening statement said at the beginning of each EFT treatment that defines and helps neutralize the problem. In EFT, the standard Setup Phrase is "Even though I have this _____, I fully and completely accept myself."

Story Technique, or Tell the Story Technique. Narrate or tell out loud the story of a specific event dealing with trauma, grief, anger, and so on, and stop to tap whenever the story becomes emotionally intense. Each of the stopping points represents another aspect of the issue that, on occasion, will take you to even deeper issues. This technique is similar to the Movie Technique, except that in the Movie Technique, you simply watch past events unfold in your mind. In the Story Technique, you describe them out loud.

Surrogate or Proxy Tapping. Tapping on yourself on behalf of another person. The person can be present or not. Another way to perform surrogate or proxy tapping is to substitute a photograph, picture, or line drawing for the person and tap on that.

Tail-Enders. The "yes, but" statements that create negative self-talk. When you state a goal or affirmation, tail-enders point the way to core issues.

Tearless Trauma Technique. This is another way of approaching an emotional problem in a gentle way. It involves having the client guess as to the emotional intensity of a past event rather than painfully relive it mentally.

Writings on Your Walls. Limiting beliefs and attitudes that result from cultural conditioning or family attitudes, these are often illogical and harmful yet very strong subconscious influences.

Yin and Yang. See Chi.

Appendix A:
The Full Basic Recipe

There are as many versions of EFT as there are people. However, there is one version of EFT that has been validated in more than twenty clinical trials, so we know it works. These studies can be evaluated using criteria for "empirically validated therapies" published by the Clinical Psychology division of the American Psychological Association (Chambless et al., 1996; Chambless et al., 1998; Chambless & Hollon, 1998). According to these criteria, EFT is an evidence-based practice that is effective for anxiety, depression, phobias, and posttraumatic stress disorder or PTSD (Feinstein, 2012). We call this evidence-based form Clinical EFT (Church, 2013a).

There is a long and a short version of the Basic Recipe used in Clinical EFT. The short Basic Recipe is the one used throughout this book, and it's very effective, as all those studies show. Yet it's well worth learning the long form as well. It's called the Full Basic Recipe. The reason for learning the long form is that it includes additional techniques that are useful for difficult issues. Most of the time, all you'll need is the short form of the Basic Recipe. Occasionally, you'll find that you don't make much progress that way, and you'll need the procedures in the Full Basic Recipe. It includes tapping points on the finger, as well as an eye movement protocol called the 9 Gamut Procedure.

Recent research shows that eye movements are closely linked to the brain's ability to process traumatic events (Ruden, 2005; Tym, Beaumont, & Lioulios, 2009). When a memory carries no emotional charge, you can move your eyes smoothly through your field of peripheral vision. But a traumatic memory interferes with smooth eye rotation, and the eyes skip around; it's almost as if the person doesn't want to "see" the traumatic memory again. When you use EFT's 9 Gamut Procedure, eye movements show you whether or not the traumatic memory has been resolved. It's also useful (a) when a client says they cannot remember a specific event, (b) when working with nonverbal, preverbal or pre-birth trauma, and (c) when working on a large number of traumatic events simultaneously, for instance with a client who was beaten frequently as a child. In these three cases, the 9 Gamut can produce startlingly good results where little else is effective. This makes it extremely important tool in your EFT toolkit. There are forty-eight Clinical EFT methods, which you'll find listed at the EFTUniverse.com website and summarized at ClinicalEFT.com. Familiarity with all of them is why practitioners who use Clinical EFT are so effective with a variety of clients and conditions. Clinical EFT is the method taught in *The EFT Manual* (Church, 2013b).

There are four parts to the Full Basic Recipe: The Setup, the Sequence, the 9 Gamut, and a second application of the Sequence. Here's how they're put together.

Ingredient #1: The Setup

The Full Basic Recipe begins with the Setup Phrase:

Even though I have this _____, I deeply and completely accept myself.

While reciting the Setup Phrase, either tap on the Karate Chop point or massage your Sore Spot.

The Sore Spot (described below) is not part of the shortcut EFT method described in this book, but it can be substituted for the Karate Chop point at the beginning of any EFT session. Here's how to find it.

The Sore Spot

There are two Sore Spots and it doesn't matter which one you use. They are located in the upper left and right portions of the chest.

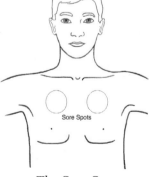

The Sore Spot.

Go to the base of the throat about where a man would knot his tie. Poke around in this area and you will find a U shaped notch at the top of your sternum (breastbone). From the top of that notch go down 2 or 3 inches toward your navel and sideways 2 or 3 inches to your left (or right). You should now be in the upper left (or right) portion of your chest. If you press vigorously in that area (within a 2-inch radius) you will find a spot that feels sore or tender. This happens because lymphatic congestion occurs there. When you rub it, you disperse that congestion. Fortunately, after a few episodes the congestion is all dispersed and the soreness goes away. Then you can rub it with no discomfort whatsoever.

I don't mean to overplay the soreness you may feel. You won't feel massive, intense pain by rubbing this Sore Spot. It is certainly bearable and should cause no undue discomfort. If it does, then lighten up your pressure a little.

Also, if you've had some kind of operation in that area of the chest or if there's any medical reason whatsoever why you shouldn't be probing around in that specific area then *switch to the other side*. Both sides are equally effective. In any case, if there is any doubt, consult your health practitioner before proceeding or simply tap the Karate Chop point instead.

Ingredient #2: The Sequence

The Sequence involves tapping on the Eyebrow, Side of Eye, Under Eye, Under Nose, Chin, Collarbone, Under Arm, and Below Nipple points.

The **Below Nipple** point is a newer addition to the full sequence. It was originally left out because it's in an awkward position for ladies while in social situations (restaurants, etc.) as well as in workshops. Even though the EFT results have been superb without it, I include it now for completeness. For men, it is one inch below the nipple. For ladies, it's where the under-skin of the breast meets the chest wall. Some call it the "underwire" point on an underwire bra. This point is abbreviated **BN** for **B**elow Nipple.

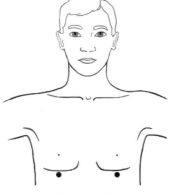

Below the Nipple (**BN**).

In addition, the Sequence in the Full Basic Recipe includes the following finger points:

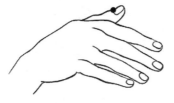

Thumb (**Th**) Point.

Thumb: On the outside edge of your thumb at a point even with the base of the thumbnail. This point is abbreviated **Th** for **Thumb.**

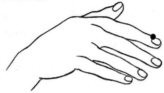

The Index Finger (**IF**) Point.

Index Finger: On the side of your index finger (the side facing your thumb) at a point even with the base of the fingernail. This point is abbreviated **IF** for Index Finger.

The Middle Finger (**MF**) Point.

Middle Finger: On the side of your middle finger (the side closest to your thumb) at a point even with the base of the fingernail. This point is abbreviated **MF** for Middle Finger.

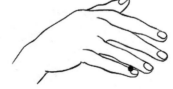

The Baby Finger (**BF**) Point.

Baby Finger: On the inside of your baby finger (the side closest to your thumb) at a point even with the base of the fingernail. This point is abbreviated **BF** for **B**aby **F**inger.

You may have noticed that the Sequence does not include the Ring Finger. However, some include it for convenience, and this does not interfere with EFT's effectiveness.

The Karate Chop (**KC**) Point.

Karate Chop: The last point is the Karate Chop point, which can also be used at the beginning of the Setup.

Thus, the complete Sequence consists of the following EFT points, which are tapped while one repeats a reminder phrase that describes the problem, such as "This headache" or "This fear of heights."

EB = Beginning of the **E**ye**B**row

SE = **S**ide of the **E**ye

UE = **U**nder the **E**ye

UN = **U**nder the **N**ose

Ch = **Ch**in

CB = Beginning of the **C**ollar**B**one

UA = **U**nder the **A**rm

BN = **B**elow the **N**ipple

Th = **Th**umb

IF = **I**ndex **F**inger

MF = **M**iddle **F**inger

BF = **B**aby **F**inger

KC = **K**arate **C**hop

Ingredient #3: The 9 Gamut Procedure

The 9 Gamut Procedure is designed to engage parts of the brain involved in the resolution of trauma. It involves eye movements, humming, and counting. It's designed to engage both the left and right sides of the brain, through counting and music. Recent research has demonstrated a link between the processing of traumatic memories and the stability of peripheral vision, and the eye movements used in the 9 Gamut take advantage of these discoveries. Clinicians report that it is very useful in removing the emotional charge of very early trauma, such as events that occurred in the first few years of life, when there are no conscious memories accessible. The 9 Gamut is also useful to clear the intensity of a large number of similar traumatic events simultaneously.

The 9 Gamut Procedure is a 10-second process in which nine "brain stimulating" actions are performed while one continuously taps on one of the body's energy points—the Gamut point. It has been found, after years of experience, that this routine can add efficiency to EFT and hasten your progress towards emotional freedom, especially when *sandwiched* between two trips through the Sequence.

One way to help memorize the Basic Recipe is to look at it as though it is a ham sandwich. The Setup is the preparation for the ham sandwich and the sandwich itself consists of two slices of bread (The Sequence) with the ham, or middle portion, as the 9 Gamut Procedure.

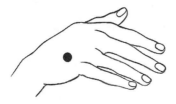

The Gamut Point.

To do the 9 Gamut Procedure, you must first locate the Gamut point. It is on the back of either hand and is 1/2 inch behind the midpoint between the knuckles at the base of the ring finger and the little finger.

If you draw an imaginary line between the knuckles at the base of the ring finger and little finger and consider that line to be the base of an equilateral triangle whose other sides converge to a point (apex) in the direction of the wrist, then the Gamut point would be located at the apex of the triangle. With the index finger of your tapping hand, feel for a small indentation on the back of your tapped hand near the base of the little finger and ring finger. There is just enough room there to tap with the tips of your index and middle fingers.

Next, you must perform nine different steps while tapping the Gamut point continuously. These 9 Gamut steps are:

1. Eyes closed.

2. Eyes open.

3. Eyes down hard right while holding the head steady.

4. Eyes down hard left while holding the head steady.

5. Roll the eyes in a circle as though your nose is at the center of a clock and you are trying to see all the numbers in order.

6. Roll the eyes in a circle in the reverse direction.

7. Hum two seconds of a song (I usually suggest "Happy Birthday").

8. Count rapidly from 1 to 5.

9. Hum two seconds of a song again.

Note that these nine actions are presented in a certain order and I suggest that you memorize them in the order given. However, you can mix the order up if you wish so long as you do all nine of them *and* you perform the last three together as a unit. That is, you hum for two seconds, then count, then hum the song again, in that order. Years of experience have proven this to be important.

Also, note that for some people humming "Happy Birthday" causes resistance because it brings up memories of unhappy birthdays. In this case, you can either use EFT on those unhappy memories and resolve them or you can side-step this issue for now by substituting some other song.

Ingredient #4: The Sequence (again)

The fourth and last ingredient in the Basic Recipe is another trip through The Sequence, including the finger points.

As in the shortcut Basic Recipe, check for any remaining discomfort, in which case you'll do another round of EFT tapping using a modified Setup Phrase:

> *Even though I still have some of this _____, I deeply and completely accept myself.*

You will add "remaining" to the Reminder Phrases as you tap through the complete Sequence.

References

Chambless, D., Baker, M. J., Baucom, D. H., Beutler, L. E., Calhoun, K. S., Crits-Christoph, P.,…Woody, S. R. (1998). Update on empirically validated therapies, II. *Clinical Psychologist, 51,* 3–16.

Chambless, D., & Hollon, S. D. (1998). Defining empirically supported therapies. *Journal of Consulting and Clinical Psychology, 66,* 7–18.

Chambless, D. L., Sanderson, W. C., Shoham, V., Bennett Johnson, S., Pope, K. S., Crits-Christoph, P.,…McCurry, C. (1996). An update on empirically validated therapies. *The Clinical Psychologist, 49,* 5–18.

Church, D. (2013a). Clinical EFT as an evidence-based practice for the treatment of psychological and physiological conditions. In *The Clinical EFT handbook, Vol 1.* (Eds. Church & Marohn). Santa Rosa, CA: Energy Psychology Press.

Church, D. (2013b). *The EFT manual* (3rd ed.). Santa Rosa, CA: Energy Psychology Press.

Feinstein, D. (2012). Acupoint stimulation in treating psychological disorders: Evidence of efficacy. *Review of General Psychology, 16,* 364–380. doi:10.1037/a0028602

Ruden, R. A. (2005). A neurological basis for the observed peripheral sensory modulation of emotional responses, *Traumatology, 11*(3), 145–158.

Tym, R., Beaumont, P., & Lioulios, T. (2009). Two persisting pathophysiological visual phenomena following psychological trauma and their elimination with rapid eye movements: A possible refinement of construct PTSD and its visual state marker. *Traumatology, 15*(3),23–33.

Appendix B:
Easy EFT

Now I would like to introduce you to a fast, effective, and effortless way to learn EFT. It's literally as easy as watching a video and tapping along with it. You can use one of the many Tap-Along Videos at www.EFTUniverse.com for this purpose. Easy EFT is a three-step process that requires no training or experience with EFT.

1. Identify the issues.

First, write up a list of troublesome symptoms, self-improvement goals, and other problems, and rate the intensity of each on a scale of 0 to 10, with 0 being no emotional intensity, and 10 being maximum intensity. Here are some examples:

Shoulder pain: 7   Performance Stress: 5   Binge Eating: 9

You can also tap for specific events that bother you, such as:

I'm mad at my coworker who swore at me last week: 8

I'm upset that my daughter was held back from third grade by the principal: 7

I hate myself for giving in to that craving and eating a tub of ice cream: 9

When my mentor criticized me, I felt so hurt: 10

2. Tap along.

As you watch the video, tap along with the coach and client. You can pick one that closely matches your issue from the dozens available on EFTUniverse.com. Even if the issue in the Tap-Along Video isn't an exact match with yours, your brain is smart enough, and eager enough to heal, that it will associate your problem with the one you're witnessing.

3. Check your results.

Revisit your list of issues and write down their new 0-to-10 intensities. You should notice some improvement each time. The more sessions you tap along with, the better your results.

It's that simple! For the best results, review the *Questions and Answers* and *Helpful Tips* that follow.

Questions and Answers about Easy EFT

Q: How was Easy EFT discovered?

A: Therapists offering EFT to their clients began to report that their issues resolved as well. They would conduct sesssions with others and discover that an illness or phobia from which they'd previously suffered had disappeared.

We then began to put this phenomenon, called Borrowing Benefits, to an experimental test. We performed several studies, and found that just watching someone else's session while tapping along produced substantial reductions in anxiety, depression, phobias, and other psychological problems (Church & Brooks, 2010; Palmer-Hoffman & Brooks, 2011; Rowe, 2005).

Q: Why does Easy EFT work so well?

A: As you tap along with the real-life people featured on our videos, a part of your brain called the hippocampus finds similarities between your issues and the ones being addressed in the session. We also have "mirror neurons" in our brains that fire as we watch a similar experience being enacted by someone else. Mirror neurons mimic the other person's experience in our own brains.

Q: Can I really benefit from a session that deals with someone else's issue?

A: Yes. We're empathetically wired to other human beings; the ability to recognize and respond to the emotions of others is a valuable evolutionary skill. You needn't have the same experience to benefit. Just as you laugh or cry (have an emotional reaction) during a movie in which the characters are having experiences nothing like yours, your brain responds to the emotions of those you watch. You can tell if you are making progress by recording your SUD score regularly.

Q: What should I expect?

A: Your results may be dramatic improvement, incremental improvement, or no improvement. Studies suggest that substantial improvement, though not complete remission, is the norm.

Q: Are there any cautions regarding this process?

A: While Easy EFT is relatively gentle and most people experience benefits, you might feel emotional or physical stress. With EFT as with any other healing method, you should always consult your primary care provider in advance.

Helpful Tips for Getting the Most out of Easy EFT

Watch the Tap-Along Videos at EFT Universe. This will acquaint you with the basic tapping points and make it easier for you to tap along.

- You do not have to read *The EFT Manual* (Church, 2013) to benefit from Easy EFT.

- You may find that the EFT sessions vary the pace and order of the points tapped. Just follow along and don't worry about these variations.

- **At first, you may find the tapping pace in the sessions to be too fast for you to follow along.** That's okay, just do your best. The process can still help you even if you miss a tapping point here or there. Eventually, you will get used to the process and the pace will be easy to follow.

Give careful consideration to your list of issues and their 0-to-10 intensities because tracking your progress is essential to understanding the power of EFT.

- For your list, go back to childhood and write down a list of events that elicited negative emotions such as anger, guilt, and shame. Give each a SUD score of 0 to 10. Also list body sensations such as pain and score them the same way.

- If you can't find a 0-to-10 intensity, that's okay. Just estimate what the number should be. The mere fact that you remembered an issue means you have some sort of charge on it, though you might not be fully in touch with it.

- List as many issues as you want. This gives you an opportunity to determine if, as you tap on one, others diminish in intensity. The generalization effect can simulaneously reduce the charge around a number of events.

- Your list might look something like the spreadsheet below after a few tap-along sessions. This example is for illustration only and does not indicate what you should expect for the specific items listed. You might find the intensity of some issues dropping more rapidly than others.

Issue	Original 0-to-10	Session 1 0-to-10	Session 2 0-to-10	Session 3 0-to-10	Etc.
Fear of Heights	8	5	2	3	
Easily Angered	10	10	5	2	
Test Anxiety	7	7	5	7	
Knee Pain	9	2	0	0	
Digestion Problems	4	4	2	3	
Etc.					

Some of your results may be subtle and you may not notice them until later. You may also experience some pleasant "side benefits" and discover improvements that you weren't expecting. Here are some examples:

Uncle Joe's aggressive personality may no longer bother you.

You're no longer irritated by Aunt Peg's overbearing manner.

Your friends notice and comment on your reduced stress level.

You notice yourself scoring better at basketball.

Your insomnia is markedly improved.

You find yourself looking forward to each day's work.

Troublesome memories from your childhood may lose their sting.

Physical symptoms may improve.

Read your list of issues before each tap-along session just to remind your brain what you are working on. After that, put the list aside and just tap along and enjoy the session while Easy EFT goes to work.

Revisit your list after each tap-along session. Then go through each issue and carefully assess any changes in current intensity. Write them all down, even those that haven't changed. Then do another tap-along session and visit the list again.

Do your sessions on any schedule you like. You can do them daily, weekly, or at any time interval you choose. You can even do several per day or break them up so that you do a half session today and finish it tomorrow. It all depends on your schedule.

Work with a variety of Tap-Along Videos. There are many different issues represented in this collection, and you can experiment with a varied selection.

Make friends in the Weight Loss Discussion Group. You'll find many relevant topics in the discussion group at EFT Universe. You can ask your question and tap the rich vein of wisdom offered in the group.

Most important…have fun with it!

EFT doesn't have to be complicated, difficult, or totally serious. You'll find plenty to laugh about in our EFT books, at EFT workshops, and your own EFT sessions at home.

For books, classes, practitioners, tutorials, discussion groups, case histories, and Tap-Along Videos, visit www. EFTUniverse.com. While there, download our free EFT starter kit, and sign up for our Weekly Health Report.

References

Church, D. (2013). *The EFT manual* (3rd ed.). Santa Rosa, CA: Energy Psychology Press.

Church, D., & Brooks, A. J. (2010). The effect of a brief EFT (Emotional Freedom Techniques) self-intervention on anxiety, depression, pain and cravings in healthcare workers. *Integrative Medicine: A Clinician's Journal, 9*(4), 40–44.

Palmer-Hoffman, J., & Brooks, A. J. (2011). Psychological symptom change after group application of Emotional

Freedom Techniques (EFT). *Energy Psychology: Theory, Research, & Treatment, 5*(1), 33–38.

Rowe, J. E. (2005). The effects of EFT on long-term psychological symptoms. *Counseling and Clinical Psychology, 2,* 104–111.

Appendix C: Skinny Genes: The Online EFT Weight Loss Program

Skinny Genes is a six-week online program that combines the best practices of EFT for weight loss, as well as proven scientific methods for releasing weight and keeping it off forever. Two clinical trials have now shown that, after an EFT weight loss program, not only do participants significantly reduce their cravings, but they lose weight naturally over the course of the following six to twelve months. Other research into fad diets show that, two years after a diet, people gain back all the weight they lose, and more. EFT is the only method we are aware of in which people not only lose weight on the program, but they lose weight after the program as well.

Developed by Dawson Church and Brittany Watkins in conjunction with a behavioral scientist, the Skinny Genes weight loss program implements a step-by-step formula designed to help you overcome food cravings and eliminate their underlying emotional causes.

Over the six weeks, the goal of Skinny Genes is literally to rewire the neural network of your brain as it processes information regarding food and emotions. This neural repatterning is designed to calm anxiety and eliminate the emotional urge for food. Many participants report regaining a sense of choice: They can look at their favorite plate and take it or leave it.

The program includes audio and video lessons, as well as written PDF lessons. These train you in new concepts, methodologies, and ways of thinking with regard to your food and your life. You also receive daily action steps demonstrating new behaviors that can produce dramatic results. The program also includes monthly live coaching calls with Dawson and Skinny Genes guest coaches.

Register at www.SkinnyGenesFit.com

EFT Resources

For information about EFT, including a free downloadable Get Started package, go to www.EFTUniverse.com. On this website, you'll find thousands of case histories of people who've used EFT successfully for every conceivable problem. You'll also find practitioner listings, tutorials, books, DVDs, classes, volunteer opportunities, and other resources to allow you to get the most from EFT.

Index

A world of wellness at your fingertips!

To see more books in this series of authorized EFT guides, including...

The EFT Manual
EFT for Fibromyalgia and Chronic Fatigue
EFT for the Highly Sensitive Temperament
EFT for Sports Performance
EFT for Golf
EFT for Love Relationships
EFT for Abundance
EFT for PTSD
EFT for Procrastination
EFT for Back Pain

...go to www.EFTUniverse.com

Tapping Plan for Weight Loss

Morning:
- Review my eating plan for the day while tapping continuously.
- Weigh myself while tapping.
- Look at myself in the mirror, tapping and saying five times, "I deeply and completely accept myself."
- Review my exercise plan for the day while tapping continuously.

Daily:
- Tap immediately after any negative interaction with another person till my SUD is 2 or less.
- Whenever I recall any negative past event, do three rounds of EFT.
- Whenever I catch myself in a piece of negative self-talk, tap till my SUD is 2 or less.
- Tap continuously whenever I see or smell a food that triggers a craving.
- Tap mentally or physically while exercising.

Before Each Meal:
- Notice body sensations and tap continuously.
- Look at and smell the food while tapping three times.
- If there's a food I crave, tap five times.

During Each Meal:
- After the first three mouthfuls, pause, and do a round of EFT.
- If there's a food I crave, tap continuously while eating it.
- When there's some food left and I'm not sure whether to finish it, tap.
- When I'm finished, look at my plate and tap three rounds of EFT.

When I Slip:
- Tap continuously while saying, "I forgive myself. Even though I slipped, I deeply and completely accept myself."
- Notice any body sensations, and tap till they have a SUD of 2 or less.
- Notice any self-talk, and tap till the SUD is 2 or less.

Evening:
- Review what I ate and my experiences with tapping, while tapping continuously.
- For any negative events from earlier in my life that I recalled today, tap till SUD is 2 or less.
- Tap for, "I fall asleep quickly and easily, and sleep soundly through the night. I lose weight while I sleep. I wake up in the morning feeling completely refreshed."

EFT on a Page

1. **Where in your body** do you feel the emotional issue most strongly?

2. **Determine the distress level** in that place in your body on a scale of 0 to 10, where 10 is maximum intensity and 0 is no intensity:

   10, 9, 8, 7, 6, 5, 4, 3, 2, 1, 0

3. **The Setup:** Repeat this statement three times, while continuously tapping the Karate Chop point on the side of the hand (large dot on hand diagram below):

   "Even though I have _____ (name the problem), I deeply and completely accept myself."

4. **The Tapping Sequence:** Tap about 7 times on each of the energy points in these 2 diagrams, while repeating a brief phrase that reminds you of the problem.

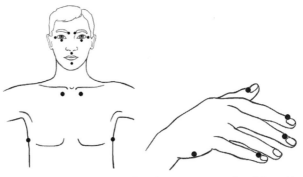

5. **Determine your distress level** again on a scale of 0 to 10 again. **If it's still high, say:**

   "Even though I have some remaining _____ (problem), I deeply and completely accept myself."

6. **Repeat from Step 1** till your distress level is as close to 0 as possible.

Find dozens of Tap-Along Videos at EFTUniverse.com